D0183194

Introducing
Beauty Therapy

Samantha Taylor

www.heinemann.co.uk

✓ Free online support
✓ Useful weblinks
✓ 24 hour online ordering

01865 888058

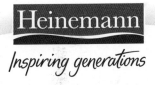

Heinemann

Inspiring generations

Heinemann is an imprint of Pearson Education Limited, a company incorporated in England and Wales, having it's registered office at Edinburgh Gate, Harlow, Essex, CM20 2JE. Registered company number: 872828

www.heinemann.co.uk

Heinemann is the registered trademark of Pearson Education Limited

© text Samantha Taylor, 2004

First published 2004

09 08
10 9 8 7

British Library Cataloguing in Publication Data is available from the British Library on request.

ISBN: 978 0 435451 39 4

Designed by Carolyn Gibson

Produced by Bridge Creative Services Limited, Bicester, Oxon

Original illustrations © Harcourt Education Limited, 2004

Illustrated by Phil Burrows and Darren Lingard

Printed in Italy by Printer Trento S.r.l

Cover photo © Getty images/Stone and Photonica/Keisen Lin

Contents

Acknowledgements

Every effort has been made to contact copyright holders of material reproduced in this book. Any omissions will be rectified in subsequent printings if notice is given to the publishers.

Every effort has been made to ensure that the information contained is valid, current and reliable. Any inaccuracies or omissions will be rectified in subsequent editions.

Thanks to my family for putting up with me always being busy! Thanks also to my family and friends for providing a support network for school pick-ups and childcare when I needed the time. This book would not have been possible without all your help.

I would like to extend my thanks to Sian Cound and her students at Abingdon and Witney College for their assistance and patience in facilitating the photo shoot; also my friend Louise for standing in for me in the photos.

Thanks to Gareth and Tony our photographers who provided a sense of humour as well as excellent photos!

Thank you to all at Heinemann for their hard work and input; particularly Pen Gresford for believing in me and Gillian Burrell for all her hard work.

Thanks also to Tiffany Tarrant at HABIA for always answering my questions when I phoned.

Samantha Taylor

Use of HABIA unit titles and element headings by kind permission of HABIA, Fraser House, Nether Hall Road, Doncaster, South Yorkshire, DN1 2PH, Tel 01302 380000, Fax 01302 380028, Email: enquiries@habia.org.uk, Website: www.habia.org.uk

We are pleased that this book has been approved by the Federation of Holistic Therapists, www.fht.org.uk.

The author and publisher would like to thank the following for permission to reproduce photographs:

Gareth Boden – pages 20, 28, 45, 53, 104; Harcourt Education/Gareth Boden – pages 79, 83, 97, 100 (bottom), 103, 107, 110, 111, 115, 116, 119, 123, 135, 139, 140, 142, 147, 148, 149, 151, 152, 153, 157; Harcourt Education/Pete Morris – pages 142, 143, 144; Daniel Lee – page 55; Lidos Salon – pages 52, 55; Mediscan – page 92; Rex Features – page 130; Science Photo Library – pages 92, 99 (bottom right), 136 (bottom left), (bottom right), (middle right), (top left), (top middle), (top right); Science Photo Library/ Dr. P Marazzi – pages 99 (bottom middle), (top left), (top right), (bottom left), 100 (right), 136 (bottom middle); Science Photo Library/ Jane Shemilt – pages 100 (left), 136 (middle); Science Photo Library/ St Bartholomew's Hospital – page 99 (top middle).

Section 1
ABOUT BEAUTY THERAPY

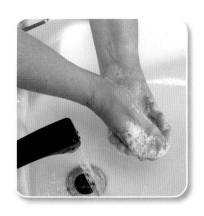 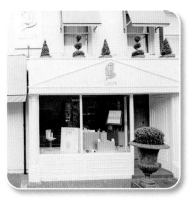 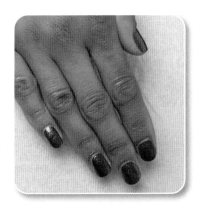

About this book

Introducing Beauty Therapy will introduce you to the basics of beauty therapy and covers all the necessary performance and criteria statements for NVQ1 Beauty Therapy. It has been written to the new standards for 2003.

Different features of this book

As you read through this book you will come across different features which will support your learning. These include:

- **Information boxes** – helpful information about good practice.
- **Check it out activities** – activities to do as projects, homework, discussions or group work.
- **Think about it boxes** – helpful hints and suggestions which will be useful in the workplace.
- **Remember boxes** – reminders of something important – often a handy tip about keeping safe in the workplace.
- **Salon stories** – examples of real-life situations that could happen in a salon.
- **Memory joggers** – questions at the end of each unit to help you recall information and show what you have learned.

In the practical skills units, you will come across different headings. These tell you about the type of information you will learn. They include:

- **Tech tools** – information about the tools that you will need to carry out a treatment.
- **Face basics** and **Nail basics** – information about the equipment you will need on your trolley or in your workspace, so that you can carry out a treatment.
- **Lotions and Potions** – information about the products needed to carry out your treatment, for example, nail varnishes, hand creams and cleansers.

What is an NVQ/SVQ?

NVQ/SVQs are qualifications that are based on the skills and knowledge that you will need at work. All NVQ/SVQs have the same structure, which includes:

- evidence
- elements
- units
- performance criteria
- range statements
- knowledge and understanding.

All of these need to be gathered in a portfolio to show proof of your learning and progress.

When studying for your NVQ, you will come across words that are used to describe parts of your learning and qualification.

What do these words mean?

- **Portfolio**

Facts and information that are collected in order to prove something.

A portfolio is a collection of *evidence* from lots of different sources. It is usually a file containing important information to show your learning. You will gather and display in your portfolio what you have learnt in order to pass your NVQ/SVQ. It can be any shape and size, as long as all the necessary evidence is included.

INFORMATION

Points to think about when putting your portfolio together

1. Does it have an attractive front cover, e.g. magazine cuttings, clear bold writing, and lots of colour and design?
2. Does it have an organised, easy-to-understand contents page and clear page numbers throughout?
3. Does it contain clear and neat notes from each lesson, either handwritten or word-processed?
4. Does it include interesting articles on Health and Beauty subjects?
5. Does it contain a conclusion – your comments at the end of the portfolio on:
   - what you learnt or gained from the course
   - how much you enjoyed the course
   - whether you are intending to progress further to Level 2
   - any other information you think might be useful?

Evidence

Evidence is proof of your learning. It can be coursework, assignments, client letters, drawings, photos or tutor comments. Most evidence will be signed by your tutor, to confirm that it is correct and your own work.

Unit

This is the subject that you will be learning about. For example, when learning about reception skills for Level 1, the unit is called: *Unit G2: Assist with salon reception duties*.

Element

Each unit or subject is made up of elements or parts. For example, Unit G2: Assist with salon reception duties contains three elements: *Maintain the reception area; Attend to clients and enquiries; Help to make appointments for salon services*.

Performance criteria

This describes what activities, either theory or practical, need to be carried out by you in order to complete the unit successfully.

Range statements

These are the situations that must be covered in your learning, for example, the type of client, type of treatment or booking method (e.g. phone or face to face).

Knowledge and understanding

This is the background knowledge that you must know so that you can carry out the treatment or activity competently.

There are 5 mandatory units that must be completed to achieve the qualification.

Unit Ref	Unit Title	Elements
G1	Ensure your own actions reduce risks to health and safety	1 Identify the hazards and evaluate the risks in your workplace 2 Reduce the risks to health and safety in your workplace
G2	Assist with salon reception duties	1 Maintain the reception area 2 Attend to clients and enquiries 3 Help to make appointments for salon services
BT1	Prepare and maintain the beauty therapy work area	1 Prepare the beauty therapy work area 2 Maintain the beauty therapy work area
BT2	Assist with facial treatments	1 Prepare for facial treatments 2 Carry out facial treatments 3 Complete the treatments
BT3	Assist with nail treatments on the hands	1 Prepare for nail treatments 2 Carry out nail treatments 3 Complete the treatments

Words and their meaning

The meaning of the word will be written in the margin, near the word in italics.

As you read through this book, you will see some words in *italic* – sloping to the side and written in colour. These are words that you may find difficult to understand, or that you need to know for beauty therapy. When you see a word like this, look in the margin at the edge of the page – there you will find the meaning of that word explained.

 CHECK IT OUT

Copy the table below. As you come across the words in italics, write the word and its meaning in the table.

You should also write down any extra words you are unsure of, then look up their meaning in a dictionary or ask your tutor.

Words	Meaning

Your career in beauty therapy

So you want to be a beauty therapist?

If you are thinking about a career in beauty therapy, you could be carrying out your skills while cruising the world on a luxury liner, working as a make-up artist, or running your own beauty salon business. What other career can offer you fun, a chance to travel the world, constant education and even the chance of fame and wealth?

The opportunities in the beauty industry are amazing, however, you must be prepared to work hard and show dedication to the industry. If you are ready to do this, you will have the opportunity for new and exciting experiences.

What makes a good beauty therapist?

- If you care about:
  - people's comfort and wellbeing
  - helping others
  - your appearance
  - your health.
- If you are:
  - kind and considerate
  - patient and understanding
  - friendly.
- If you have:
  - a strong back
  - good health.
- If you can:
  - get on well with all sorts of people whatever their age, personality or background
  - keep calm under pressure
  - remain cheerful, even when you are having a bad day or have problems at home
  - make a difference!

Then you are the right person for the job!

A healthy lifestyle

Do you realise the benefits of a healthy lifestyle? In order to stay in top condition, our body needs:

- a good balanced diet and regular meals, with healthy low fat snacks in-between to boost energy levels
- fresh air and regular exercise
- lots of water to flush out toxins
- plenty of sleep to allow the body to rest and repair itself.

If you take care of yourself, you will:

- have hair that glistens and shines instead of being dull and lifeless
- have skin that is smooth and clear, instead of spotty and greasy or dry and flaky
- be bright and enthusiastic for the day ahead, instead of feeling tired and depressed
- have patience and understanding, instead of being bad tempered and impatient
- have energy and staying power instead of having dizzy spells and feeling weak.

Losing weight the healthy way

The rate at which you burn up food for energy.

If you are constantly dieting on and off, then your body won't know when to expect its next balanced meal. When this happens, the body protects itself by storing food as fat and lowering your *metabolism*. This prevents you from losing weight successfully. And if you do lose weight, it is piled back on again quickly, as soon as you start to eat larger meals.

If you really want to lose weight, the only safe and successful way is to eat a balanced diet that contains lots of fresh fruit and vegetables, proteins, carbohydrates and not too much fat, sugar or *processed foods*.

Ready-made meals and takeaways, which contain high levels of salt, sugar and fat.

Blood sugar levels

If you go for long periods without eating, the sugar levels in your blood will fall and this will make you feel dizzy and shaky. When this happens, it is very tempting to reach for a quick fix of sugar, for example, a chocolate bar, to make you feel better. The trouble is that it only gives you a quick rush of energy, and then your sugar levels drop again. Furthermore, you've just eaten a really unhealthy, high calorie snack, and you're soon hungry again.

 CHECK IT OUT

In groups, chat to your tutor and decide what foods would be better to snack on during the day.
Then discuss your eating habits. Are they good or bad?

INFORMATION

- Too much sunbathing can dry out your skin and hair, and cause your skin to age early.
- Smoking can cause your skin to become sensitive, red and blotchy. The tobacco and nicotine in cigarettes also use up important vitamins and minerals that help the body to work well.
- Exercise, fresh air and plenty of sleep are necessary if you want to be happy, healthy and fit. Don't think that years of bad treatment of your body won't affect your health in the long-run.

In the beauty industry, clients will look to you for your skills and expertise. You will be asked for advice and guidance, and while it is up to the client to choose what advice she follows, remember that your bad habits will show in your eyes, skin, nails and general health. So it is important that you practise what you recommend.

Section 2
IN THE WORKPLACE

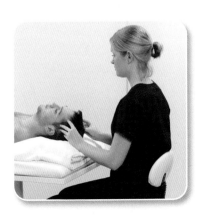
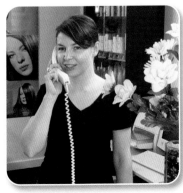
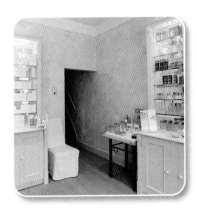

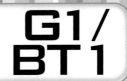
Introduction

The Beauty Industry hasn't always been taken as seriously as it is now – it has taken many years for it to win the respect it deserves. Excellent training and high standards have improved its reputation and this now means that the Beauty Industry is recognised as providing an important service to the public. The knowledge and skills needed within the industry are broad and various. Beauty therapists should therefore take care not to allow their professional standards to slip.

Units such as this one covering health and safety regulations, may not be a favourite topic – we all prefer to learn about the practical side. However, the Beauty Industry would suffer if we did not show the highest standards of *health*, *safety* and *hygiene* at all times.

Health = fitness and wellbeing
Safety = not dangerous
Hygiene = cleanliness

High standards of health, safety and hygiene prevent:

- dirty salons and messy staff
- dangerous work areas
- use of unsafe equipment
- illness and cross-infection
- accidents and injury
- a very poor *reputation*.

The name, praise or criticism the salon earns for itself.

Every workplace, whether a shop, office, factory or beauty salon, must follow a set of health and safety rules laid down by the *Health and Safety Executive* (HSE). This legislation is designed to protect both employers and employees from accident, illness and injury.

Laws affecting the running of the business, treatment, premises, environment and employees.

INFORMATION

It's a fact that accidents in the home and at work are increasing. It will never be possible to prevent accidents from happening completely, but if everyone does their bit at work to cut down the risks, the workplace will be a much safer place.

In this unit, you will cover the following topics:

- staying safe in the workplace
- rules and regulations
- salon hygiene
- comfort controls
- insurance
- security and safekeeping.

Stay safe!

What you will learn about:
- The Health and Safety at Work Act 1974
- Hazards and risks
- Spotting hazards
- Reporting accidents
- First Aid

The Health and Safety at Work Act 1974

Responsibility according to the law.

This Act is the main law-making information for employers and employees, all of whom have a *legal duty* to make sure that everyone is kept healthy, safe and well at work.

Under this Act, there are many rules and guidelines dealing with all areas of health and safety in the workplace. You do not need to know about every single one for Level 1 — those that are important to you at this stage are covered in the section on **Rules and Regulations**.

Workplace policies and codes of practice

As well as following the Health and Safety at Work Act, your workplace will have its own rules and guidelines for keeping employees and the general public safe. These are called **Workplace policies** or **codes of practice**.

It is the employer's duty to provide a safe environment for employees. In addition, employees have a duty to co-operate with the workplace policies in order to demonstrate expected standards of behaviour, and to make the salon a safer and healthier place to work.

This also includes ensuring that the salon is a non-smoking environment, as smoking affects the level of fresh air in the salon and makes it smell unpleasant. Even if staff have a cigarette outside during a break, the smell remains on their clothes and breath and can be smelt by clients during their treatment. An alcohol and drug free workplace is also essential. Any member of staff under the influence of drugs or alcohol cannot use equipment and products safely and could put others at risk. If clients are under the influence of drugs or alcohol, they will be asked to leave by the supervisor or *relevant person*.

An individual responsible for supervising work or the person you usually report to.

CHECK IT OUT

Design an information sheet that lists all the important people who are responsible for safety in your salon. For example:

1 The name of the first aider(s) and the days on which they work.

2 The name of the salon manager or supervisor who is generally responsible for help and advice in the salon.

3 The following information about the person in charge of health and safety for your salon:

- their first name and surname
- the days/hours he or she works and who is responsible if that person is away
- his or her telephone number and/or place of contact.

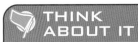

THINK ABOUT IT

It is important that you know who you must report hazards, risks, accidents, illnesses and injury to. You will need to make sure that you are familiar with these people at the beginning of your work experience and employment.

Your health and safety responsibilities at work include making sure that your actions:

1 keep you and others safe and healthy

2 follow the law

3 follow your workplace *policies*.

Rules and guidelines.

If the Health and Safety at Work Act 1974 is not followed:

- the salon could be shut down
- you or the salon could be *fined*
- the employer or member of staff could go to prison (in very serious cases).

A charge or payment as a punishment.

REMEMBER

All workplaces have their own rules and procedures that staff must follow. These are called organisational requirements.

If an employee does not follow the workplace policies on health and safety:

- there could be loss of business
- the business could get a bad reputation

- the employee could lose his or her job
- people could become ill or injured.

CHECK IT OUT

If you are doing work experience or have a Saturday job, find out your employer's workplace policies and write them down.

Your employer has a duty under the law to ensure, so far as is reasonably practicable, your health, safety and welfare at work.

Your employer must consult you or your safety representative on matters relating to your health and safety at work, including:

- any change which may substantially affect your health and safety at work, eg in procedures, equipment or ways of working;
- the employer's arrangements for getting competent people to help him/her satisfy health and safety laws;
- the information you have to be given on the likely risks and dangers arising from your work, measures to reduce or get rid of these risks and what you should do if you have to deal with a risk or danger;
- the planning of health and safety; and
- the health and safety consequences of introducing new technology.

In general, your employer's duties include:

- making your workplace safe and without risks to health;
- ensuring plant and machinery are safe and that safe systems of work are set and followed;
- ensuring articles and substances are moved, stored and used safely;
- providing adequate welfare facilities;
- giving you the information, instruction, training and supervision necessary for your health and safety.

In particular, your employer must:

- **assess the risks** to your health and safety;
- **make arrangements** for implementing the health and safety measures identified as being necessary by the assessment;
- if there are five or more employees, **record the significant findings** of the risk assessment and the arrangements for health and safety measures;
- if there are five or more employees, **draw up a health and safety policy statement**, including the health and safety organisation and arrangements in force, and **bring it to your attention.**
- **appoint someone competent** to assist with health and safety responsibilities, and consult you or your safety representative about this appointment;

- co-operate on health and safety with other employers sharing the same workplace;
- set up **emergency procedures**;
- **provide adequate first-aid facilities**;
- make sure that the **workplace** satisfies **health, safety and welfare** requirements, eg for ventilation, temperature, lighting, and sanitary, washing and rest facilities;
- make sure that **work equipment is suitable** for its intended use, so far as health and safety is concerned, and that it is **properly maintained and used**;
- **prevent or adequately control exposure** to substances which may damage your health;
- **take precautions** against danger from flammable or explosive hazards, electrical equipment, noise and radiation;
- **avoid hazardous manual handling operations**, and where they cannot be avoided, reduce the risk of injury;
- provide **health surveillance as appropriate**;
- **provide free any protective clothing or equipment**, where risks are not adequately controlled by other means;
- ensure that appropriate **safety signs are provided and maintained**;
- **report** certain, injuries, diseases and dangerous occurrences to the appropriate health and safety enforcing authority (see box below for who this is).

As an employee you have legal duties too. They include:

- **taking reasonable care** for your own health and safety and that of others who may be affected by what you do or do not do;
- **co-operating with your employer** on health and safety;
- **correctly using work items** provided by your employer, including personal protective equipment, in accordance with training or instructions; and
- **not interfering with or misusing anything provided for your health, safety or welfare.**

You can get advice on general fire precautions etc from the Fire Brigade or your fire officer.

Health and safety regulations

Hazards and risks

In the workplace, many things can cause accidents, injury or illness if they are not recognised and made safe. You will need to be able to spot these things and take steps to make sure that they do not cause a problem to you, your clients and other staff.

What is a hazard?

A hazard is a thing that could cause an accident or injury.

What is a risk?

This is the threat of something dangerous happening because of the hazard.

For example, a skincare delivery has arrived and the boxes are left lying around reception.

- The hazard would be the boxes left in the way.
- The risk is the chance that someone could trip over them and hurt him or herself.

How staff can help

There is a saying, 'an accident waiting to happen'. This means that there is a hazard that is likely to cause an injury or accident if it is not made safe. All staff must look out for these hazards at all times.

Below is a table giving you examples of hazards and the risks involved.

HAZARD	RISK
Rushing about too much, without concentrating	Bumping into people and causing an injury
Badly fitting carpet or lino	Tripping up
Highly polished floors	Slipping
Trolleys and desks overloaded with equipment and products	Furniture tipping over
A light bulb that has blown	Accidents because of poor light
A therapist carrying tools in the pocket of her uniform	Cuts or wounds if someone bumps into her
Carrying too much at once	Can't see where you are going which results in an accident or a bad back
Electrical leads trailing on the floor	Tripping over leads
Plugs that have loose or frayed leads	Possible electric shock or risk of fire
Breakages or spills that are not cleared up instantly	Cuts or slipping over
Unsterilised tools	Cross infection

Hazards and risks in the salon

 CHECK IT OUT

- In pairs, think up some hazards and risks that could arise during facial and nail treatments.
  Choose one person to think of the hazards; the other person has to say what the risks could be.

- Read the table of hazards and risks above. For each situation, state how you would make it safer and less likely to turn into an accident or injury.

Spotting hazards

 CHECK IT OUT

How good are you at spotting a hazard? Look at the poster below and write down as many hazards as you can.

Can you spot the hazards?

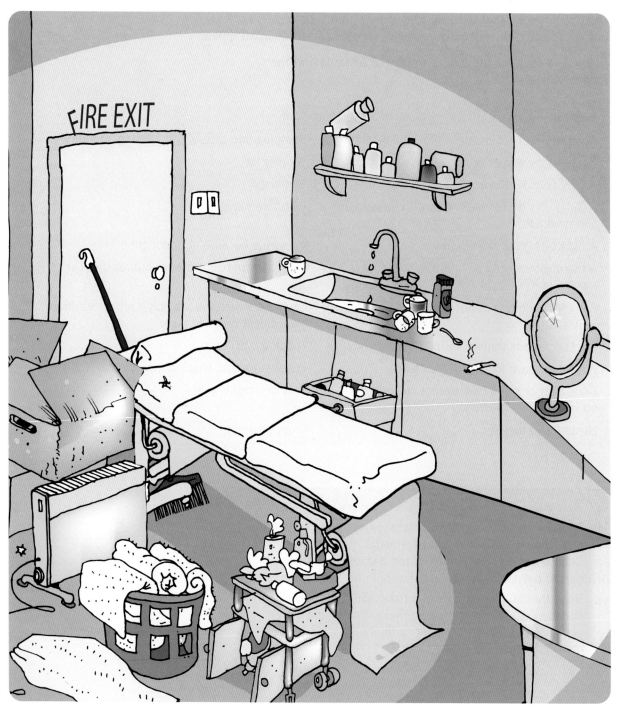

How many hazards did you spot?

Reporting accidents

All accidents and injuries must be reported to the relevant person. If a workplace employs more than 10 staff then by law it must have an **accident book**. This can be bought from a stationery shop and must be kept somewhere that is easy for all staff to access. The data protection law states that an employee's information must be kept secure and private. Therefore once the completed sheet is removed from the accident book it should be passed to the relevant person to be filed in a lockable cabinet. If your salon is small with less than 10 employees, it is still a good idea for the employer to keep a record of all accidents and injuries.

The information that should be included when reporting an accident is:

- the date and time it happened
- the place/area
- the type of accident, for example, a cut, a fall or a bang on the head, and how it happened
- the name of the injured or ill person
- what first aid was given, if any
- what happened after the accident – whether the person went to hospital, was sent home or returned to work
- the name and signature of the first aider or person who sorted the matter out.

It is *not* your responsibility to deal with accidents or give first aid. However, you *must* report to your health and safety *supervisor* anything that you think might be a danger to the general public and staff. So make sure you know who your supervisor is.

The senior member of staff to who you need to report hazards and accidents.

 REMEMBER

If you need to report an accident, act cool and calm and think very carefully about what you need to do.

First aid

The **Health and Safety Regulations (First Aid) 1981** tell employers what they must do to help prevent accidents, and how to deal with accidents when they happen. The employer *must* follow their rules and guidelines.

The main requirements are:

- a suitably stocked first aid box
- an appointed person to take care of first aid arrangements.

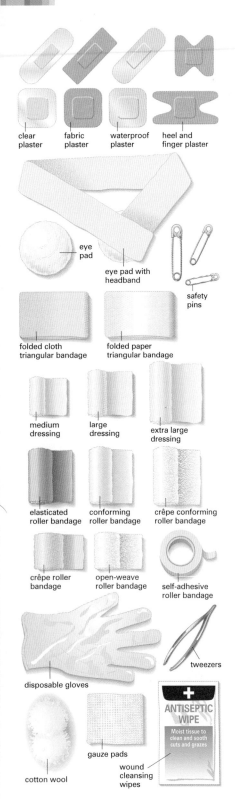

clear plaster | fabric plaster | waterproof plaster | heel and finger plaster

eye pad

eye pad with headband

safety pins

folded cloth triangular bandage | folded paper triangular bandage

medium dressing | large dressing | extra large dressing

elasticated roller bandage | conforming roller bandage | crêpe conforming roller bandage

crêpe roller bandage | open-weave roller bandage | self-adhesive roller bandage

disposable gloves

tweezers

cotton wool | gauze pads | wound cleansing wipes

The contents of a first aid box

What is first aid?

- First aid is the first help given to someone with an injury or who has become ill. It is the treatment given before the person receives professional medical aid.
- First aid includes calling for help or telephoning for an ambulance (if the problem is serious).

First aid *does not* include:

- giving medicines or tablets
- moving a person who has fallen and could possibly have broken bones – his or her injury could be made worse.

The Health and Safety Regulations 1981 state that there should be a member of staff who is trained in first aid. Once this person has been trained, he or she is qualified for three years. After this time, the person will need to re-train.

It is the job of the first aider to try to prevent a *casualty* from becoming worse before the ambulance or doctor arrives.

A person who is injured in an accident.

Important things to remember when dealing with a casualty are:

- stay calm
- listen to the person and talk quietly to him or her
- be gentle and caring
- move the casualty as little as possible
- keep the person warm with a blanket, but do not allow him or her to get too hot.

The first aid box

A first aid kit must be in a proper first aid box. This is a green box with a white cross on the front. A first aid kit must not be kept in any old container such as a biscuit tin or shoe box.

The first aid box must be kept in a place where all staff can access it easily. It should not be hidden from view, and must be labelled clearly.

The first aid box must only contain items that a first aider has been trained to use. It must not contain any medication.

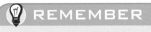

REMEMBER

First aid saves lives!

CHECK IT OUT

Think about the places that you have worked, or your school/college. Find out the following information:

- Where are the first aid boxes kept?
- Do they contain enough of the important first aid items?
- Are the contents checked regularly so that used items are replaced?

Rules and regulations

What you will learn about:

- Manual Handling Operations Regulations 1992
- Local Government (Miscellaneous Provisions) Act 1982
- Control of Substances Hazardous to Health Regulations 1999 (CoSHH)
- Fire Precaution Work Place Regulations 1997
- Electricity at Work Regulations 1989
- Gas safety (Installation and Use) Regulations 1994
- Reporting of Injuries, Diseases & Dangerous Occurrences Regulations 1995 (RIDDOR)
- Personal Protective Equipment at Work Regulations 1992
- Environmental Protection Act 1990, Waste Regulations 1992 and Special Waste Regulations 1996

Manual Handling Operations Regulations 1992

The Health and Safety Executive introduced the Manual Handling Operations Regulations in 1992 to prevent injury to the muscles and bones of the body. Injury can be caused by:

- wrong lifting methods
- poor posture
- regular and continual strain on the same part of the body
- moving objects by force that may be too heavy.

Posture, lifting and carrying

In the salon, you need to be careful how you lift and carry stock. You also need to take care over the way you sit, whether at reception or while carrying out a treatment – it is important that the chair or couch is the right height for you. To enable your body to change position regularly while working, it is better if you carry out a variety of treatments. In addition, you need to know how to hold tools correctly, and give your hands a chance to rest after a treatment.

Changeable.

It is a good idea to:

- use height *adjustable* couches and stools
- get help when carrying large, heavy or awkward things
- move and stretch your body regularly if you remain in the same position for a long time
- do exercises to keep your hands flexible.

> **REMEMBER**
>
> Always help the client on and off a treatment couch by offering your hand or arm for support and balance. After a treatment, a client might be so relaxed that he or she could easily fall off the couch. Also, if a client is not used to getting up onto a couch, he or she could misjudge its height and width.

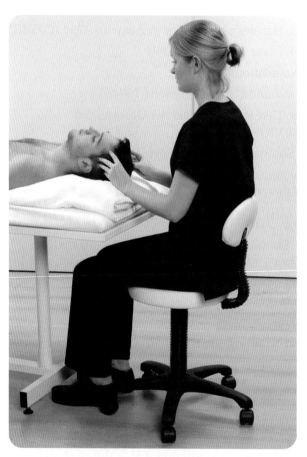

Good posture

INFORMATION

Most deliveries are brought to reception. Some are very large and heavy, and will need to be moved elsewhere before they are unpacked. It is very important that large and heavy deliveries are moved carefully, to avoid damaging you or the products.

The safe lifting method

As a beauty therapist, you will have a lifetime of bending and standing in one position and it is essential that you look after your back. The safe lifting method is shown below; make sure that you follow it.

When picking up a large or heavy item:

- bend at the knee
- use both hands to grasp the box
- use the strength in your legs to help lift the weight
- *Never* bend from the waist, as this could damage your lower back.

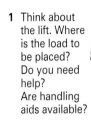 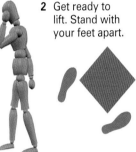 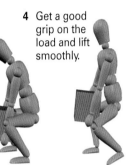 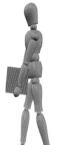 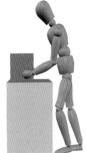

1 Think about the lift. Where is the load to be placed? Do you need help? Are handling aids available?

2 Get ready to lift. Stand with your feet apart.

3 Bend the knees. Keep the back straight. Tuck in your chin. Lean slightly forward over the load to get a good grip.

4 Get a good grip on the load and lift smoothly.

The safe lifting method

 REMEMBER

If you are unsure about whether you can lift something on your own, always get help.

If stock needs to be stored on high shelves, make sure you use a safe, non-wobbly step ladder – never use a chair.

Local Government (Miscellaneous Provisions) Act 1982

Practitioners who carry out a treatment involving the use of needles or skin piercing must register with their Local Authority. The workplace **premises** also need to be registered, unless the practitioner is **mobile**, in which case the registration will be for them only. The cost for this registration differs slightly between different authorities.

After the premises or practitioner is registered to carry out the treatments, a local authority inspector will visit to check that the levels of hygiene and safety are satisfactory. Once the checks have been satisfactorily completed, and if the practitioner is qualified, the inspector awards a certificate that allows the following treatments to be carried out:

- acupuncture
- ear and body piercing
- tattooing
- epilation.

People who practise a treatment.

A place of business.

A practitioner or therapist who travels around to carry out treatments, and does not work from one building or premises.

REMEMBER

The local council has the power to fine a business or cancel registration if hygiene is not kept to a high standard.

Control of Substances Hazardous to Health Regulations 1999 (CoSHH)

Information given by the company that makes the products or recommended safety measures

manufacturer's instructions on safety

This law requires employers to assess the risks from all harmful products and take appropriate *precautions*. All products that could be harmful must be:

- used safely and follow *safety measures*.
- stored safely
- cleaned up safely when spilt
- thrown away safely.

Employers must write down all the products they use, how they are used, stored, cleaned up and thrown away (including cleaning agents). Employers must do this because the products they use could:

Burn easily, so could cause a fire.

- be *flammable*
- be poisonous if swallowed
- cause irritation
- give out strong fumes.

Breathed in.

- be dangerous if *inhaled*
- be slippery if spilt.

A table for recording information for CoSHH

The simplest way to record information about the different products used by a salon is in a table, which is clear and easy to read. An example is given below.

Product	Hazard	Correct use	Storage	Disposal of waste	Caution
Nail varnish remover	Inhalation of flames; highly flammable.	Replace bottle tops immediately; no smoking or naked flames nearby.	Store away from direct heat in a locked cupboard, with lids fully on and bottle upright.	Do not incinerate. Dispose of by burning.	If spilt, clear up immediately as it can dissolve some plastics such as cushion flooring, and mark trolleys and equipment. If spilt on clothes, minimise the fumes by sponging with water.

CHECK IT OUT

Ask your tutor which hazardous substances are used on your course. Ask to look at the list that says how they should be handled.

REMEMBER

It is **very important** that manufacturers' instructions are followed. These are usually shown on the packaging of a product, or on a separate leaflet inside the box.
If instructions are not followed, accidents and injuries can occur. Any accidents or injuries that occur when the manufacturers' instructions are not followed, would not be covered by the salon's insurance.

Fire Precaution Work Place Regulations 1997

The law says that all workplaces must carry out a fire *risk assessment* and a yearly fire drill. All staff must be trained in the fire drill – what to do in the event of a fire and how to *evacuate* the building safely.

A formal check to discover what the dangers of fire are and what can be done to prevent a fire.

To leave a place of danger.

The fire drill

The information that staff should be given about the fire drill includes:

- how to sound the alarm and call for help
- who to report to
- the responsibilities of staff to both clients and the people they work with
- how to leave the building safely
- where the emergency exit is
- where the *assembly point* is.

An agreed meeting place outside a building.

REMEMBER

Always find out the fire and evacuation procedure for any place in which you work or study. By law, an employer, school or college must give you this information straight away. If they have not, make sure that you find out as soon as possible.

Your responsibilities at work: fire safety

Do:

- leave all doors unlocked wherever possible
- keep flammable products away from heat
- report anything that you think may be a fire hazard – it is better to be safe than sorry.

Don't:

- block doorways and exits
- smoke inside
- warm towels on electric or gas heaters.

Building evacuation procedures in the event of fire or bomb alert

The following procedure has been agreed and must be followed. Any staff member who does not comply is committing an infringement of the college disciplinary code. Whenever a fire occurs, the main consideration is to get everybody out of the building safely. Protection of personal or college property is incidental.

Raising the alarm

Anyone discovering a fire must immediately raise the alarm by operating the nearest fire alarm and report to the controller the fire location.

On hearing the alarm the receptionist will immediately contact the emergency services and then evacuate the building.

In the event of a fire being discovered when the reception is unmanned – the premises officer on duty will contact the emergency services and assume control.

On hearing the alarm

All those in senior positions proceed to the control point, normally at a main entrance to the building – where one person must take control of the proceedings.

All other staff: close windows; switch off machinery and lights, and close doors on leaving the room.

Assist less able colleagues, leave the building by the nearest marked route and proceed quickly to the appropriate assembly point. Staff must supervise their class.

Staff evacuating the building must check their locality is clear.

Assembly points

Everyone must remain at assembly points well away from buildings and clear of access roads.

Report to control in person or via two-way radios where allocated.

Everyone must remain at assembly points until further instructions.

DO NOT re-enter the building until you are told it is safe to do so.

An example of a fire and evacuation procedure

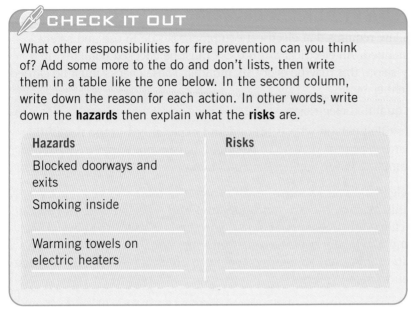

CHECK IT OUT

What other responsibilities for fire prevention can you think of? Add some more to the do and don't lists, then write them in a table like the one below. In the second column, write down the reason for each action. In other words, write down the **hazards** then explain what the **risks** are.

Hazards	Risks
Blocked doorways and exits	
Smoking inside	
Warming towels on electric heaters	

Fire extinguishers

All workplaces must have fire-fighting equipment. It should be easy to access and in good working order.

There are different *extinguishers* for different types of fire. Using a fire extinguisher is not easy and, unless you are confident that you know how and which one to use, don't try – you could put yourself or others at risk.

Extinguish means to put out or destroy. An extinguisher is a tool for doing this.

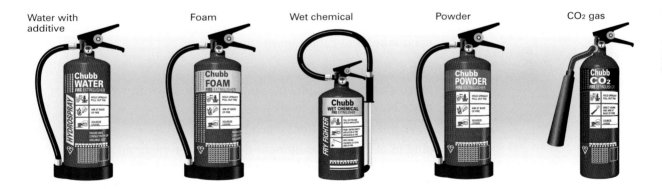

Water with additive | Foam | Wet chemical | Powder | CO_2 gas

Small fires can be put out using a fire blanket or a bucket of sand.

Different types of fire extinguishers

CHECK IT OUT

Can you think of three types of fire-fighting equipment? Describe how you would use them.

Machines and equipment.

Electricity at Work Regulations 1989

This law requires that electrical equipment is safe to use and safely maintained. All electrical *appliances* must be checked regularly. In a busy salon, this may be every six months. These checks must be carried out either by:

- a qualified electrician
- a skilled person who is trained and experienced in the use of that particular appliance, for example, a person employed by the company who supplies the equipment.

All electrical checks must be written in a book that is kept specifically for this reason. The date and signature of the person who carried out the check must be entered along with the reason for the check, for example, whether it was a repair or a just a maintenance check. In addition, information needs to be given about the exact nature of the repair or safety check.

The book must be available for inspection by the health and safety authority.

Your responsibilities at work: electrical appliances

Report to your supervisor *immediately*:

- any faulty plugs, frayed wires or loose connections
- any flickering or faulty lights.

Do:

- switch off and unplug all machines after use
- check that all equipment trolleys are stable and not on uneven floors
- wind wires and cables up neatly.

Don't:

- touch electrical equipment, plugs or switches with wet hands or place bowls of water nearby
- leave trailing wires from machines
- plug in or use any equipment that has been reported as faulty.

Gas safety (Installation and Use) Regulations 1994

Under these regulations, a workplace must allow gas and HSE inspectors to enter the premises in order to disconnect dangerous gas appliances. All gas appliances must be installed, maintained and used safely.

Your responsibilities at work:

Report to your supervisor immediately:

Feeling sick – that you are going to vomit.

- any unusual smell
- any regular headaches, *nausea* or unexplained tiredness.

Reporting of Injuries, Diseases and Dangerous Occurrences Regulations 1995 (RIDDOR)

Under these regulations, the employer must send a report to the local authority if:

- anyone dies or is seriously injured at work
- is absent from work for more than three days because of a *diagnosed* disease or accident connected with work.

Confirmed by a medical doctor or specialist.

Personal Protective Equipment at Work Regulations 1992

These regulations state that staff must have training in the use of equipment, and details the use of protective clothing for safety at work.

Your responsibilities at work

- Never use any equipment for which you have not received training.
- Always wear the recommended protective clothing.

 REMEMBER

Don't place tools in your pockets as many are pointed or sharp and could result in an injury if you fall or bump into someone.

Environmental Protection Act 1990, Waste Regulations 1992 and Special Waste Regulations 1996

These regulations state that *clinical* waste must be separated from normal waste and disposed of by *licensed incineration*.

Waste items consisting of human tissue, blood, bodily fluids, swabs, dressings, syringes or needles.

Your responsibilities at work

- Never dispose of clinical waste in a normal waste bin.

Official and permitted burning.

Keep it clean!

What you will learn about:

- Salon hygiene
- Personal hygiene
- Germ facts

Salon hygiene

These are requirements laid down by law, industry codes of practice or workplace written procedures.

Passing on infection

Infection can pass from one person to another in two ways:

Direct contact

This is when an infection passes straight from one person to another. This can occur by:

- the touching of skin
- sneezing
- coughing
- breathing.

Indirect contact

This is when infection passes from one person to another through an unclean object, for example:

- a towel
- a jar of cream
- tweezers
- a wet floor
- dirty equipment and tools.

This is called *cross-infection*.

Cross-infection is the transfer of germs and bacteria through poor hygiene.

REMEMBER

Cross-infection can take place in the salon if high standards of hygiene are not kept at all times.

Preventing cross-infection

There are three ways to make sure that the work environment is clean and germ free.

① Sanitisation

Sanitisation is cleaning or washing to promote health by reducing the growth of germs and bacteria. It also removes dust and dirt.

- When sanitising the hands, use liquid soap and paper towels as these are the most hygienic.
- Before any disinfection and sterilising, always sanitise tools and equipment by washing.
- Chemicals used for sanitising include surface agents (surfactant)s alcohols and hypochlorites.

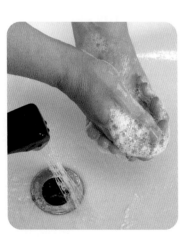

Thorough hand washing is essential to good hygiene

CHECK IT OUT

In your college or salon, look at the list of ingredients on the bottles of the products used for sanitisation.

REMEMBER

Wet hands are not clean hands. It is very important to dry them thoroughly after washing.

2 Disinfecting

Disinfection is a form of cleaning in which surfaces, trolleys and equipment are wiped over with a *disinfectant* solution.

A chemical that kills micro-organisms.

This reduces the numbers of germs and bacteria to a level that is less harmful to health. Most disinfectant solutions are alcohol or bleach based.

For treatments in which the skin must be very clean, for example, electrolysis and ear piercing, a disinfectant solution or wipe is used on the skin.

To keep previously sterilised tools clean during a treatment place them in a jar of disinfectant solution.

3 Sterilisation

Sterilisation is a cleaning method that kills all germs and bacteria. It is used for tools and equipment. The tools are placed in a very high temperature to kill all germs and bacteria.

However, if the sterilisation routine is not thorough, some germs will remain.

There are only two reliable methods of sterilisation:

- **Dry heat** sterilising, which takes place in a **hot air oven**.
- **Steam** sterilising, which takes place in an **autoclave**.

There are other methods of sterilisation:

- **Ultraviolet** sterilising, which takes place in an **ultraviolet cabinet**.
- **Heat destruction**, which takes place in a **bead steriliser**.

However, these methods are not always 100 per cent effective at reaching all the surfaces of the tools. In addition, the temperatures can vary in places, so are not always hot enough to kill the germs and bacteria.

INFORMATION

Items such as mask sponges, make-up brushes and mask brushes are very difficult to sterilise completely and can become a home for many germs. Not all salons have an autoclave or hot air oven, so it is essential that you wash them with hot soapy water then allow them to dry completely. Once you have done this, place them in a sterilising ultraviolet cabinet to reduce the number of bacteria.

The best option, however, is to use disposable brushes and sponges where possible.

REMEMBER

All disinfectants must be stored, used and disposed of following the manufacturer's instructions and CoSHH regulations.

Your responsibilities at work: cutting down the risk of infection

1. Wash and dry your hands before and after each client.
2. Always use clean towels and a protective couch roll for each client.
3. Keep your nails short with no varnish, and tie your hair back neatly.
4. Remove all jewellery.
5. Wear a clean and fresh uniform.
6. Wear a plaster on any cuts or grazes.
7. Don't eat and drink in the treatment area.
8. Never cough, sneeze or blow your nose over a client.
9. Don't carry out a treatment if you have a cold or the 'flu.
10. Use sterilised equipment only.
11. Hold sterilised tools by the handle only.
12. Wipe down surfaces and trolleys with a disinfectant solution regularly.
13. Don't share tools.
14. Use disposable tools where possible.
15. Re-sterilise any tools that have been dropped on the floor.
16. Replace tops on products straight away.
17. Always use spatulas to remove creams from jars.
18. Dust and clean the therapist's work area regularly.
19. Never treat open cuts, bites or stings.
20. Never treat anyone with a *contra-indication*.

A condition that makes the client unsuitable for treatment, for example, skin infections or high blood pressure.

REMEMBER

Disinfection and sterilisation is useless on unclean tools and equipment. Your first step must always be to sanitise them by washing!

Personal hygiene

You must always take care to ensure good personal hygiene at work. The chart on page 31 tells you what you should do to achieve this.

Action	How it improves personal hygiene
Bath or shower daily	To remove stale sweat, which will begin to smell as bacteria grows in it
Use an underarm anti-perspirant or deodorant daily	To keep you smelling fresh and to cut down on sweating
Step up your mouth hygiene! Look after your teeth and gums: ■ clean your teeth twice daily ■ floss daily ■ rinse with a mouthwash while at work	Clean teeth and gums mean fresh breath. If you continue to have a mouth odour problem then you could have a build up of old food around your teeth and gums A mouthwash will help to keep your mouth fresh and stop bacteria from growing in your mouth
Wear a clean, ironed uniform	Uniforms can easily become dirty and absorb smells in the environment, including smells from other people and body odour
Have short, neat nails with no varnish	Dirt, germs and bacteria build up under long nails. Varnish-free nails look cleaner and fresher than painted ones. Some clients can be sensitive to the ingredients in nail varnish
Wash your hands with soap and dry them thoroughly after every visit to the toilet	If you do not wash and dry your hands thoroughly, you will pass many bacteria and germs to others when you carry out a treatment
Never eat in the treatment area	Eating in the treatment area causes the spread of bacteria, and will encourage the presence of insects and disease-spreading flies
Remove jewellery when carrying out a treatment	Bacteria can build up under rings

Germ facts

Actions to ensure good personal hygiene

INFORMATION

You might think that your salon reception desk is spotless. However, looks can be deceiving. Dr Charles Gerba, an American microbiologist, carried out a study of the workplace. He found that the average office desk carries 400 times more bacteria than the average toilet seat!

■ Germs are **everywhere** – they travel fast and multiply constantly.

■ Germs grow best in warm damp conditions, so remember to clean and dry your manicure and pedicure bowls thoroughly.

■ When we cough and sneeze, germs pass through the air at high speeds.

■ To be clean, hands must be dried thoroughly after washing. If you don't dry your hands properly, the water left on your skin can help to move germs from person to person.

■ Germs gather under long or artificial nails.

- The top five germ-ridden places are:
  - the phone
  - the desktop
  - the water fountain
  - microwave door handles
  - the computer keyboard.
- Toilet seats and photocopiers are the least germ-ridden places.
- Doorknobs, pens, money, taps and your lunch are *all* covered with bacteria and viruses ready to invade you.
- A polite handshake can result in a stinking cold.
- A sanitising spray is excellent for cutting down the amount of germs in the environment.

Comfort controls

In this section, you will learn about the controls needed to make sure that the salon surroundings are comfortable, warm and clean – all the things which make sure that a salon visit is enjoyable and that the work environment is satisfying for the staff.

What you will learn about:

- What makes a clean salon
- The importance of hot and cold running water
- Lighting
- The treatment room
- A place to relax and unwind
- Fresh air
- The ideal temperature

What makes a clean salon

As a beauty therapy assistant, one of your responsibilities is to make sure that the work area is left clean, tidy and ready for the next treatment. You will also need to sanitise the tools and equipment after use, and check that they have been sterilised before the next treatment.

> **INFORMATION**
>
> If the tools have not been sterilised you must inform the senior therapist, who will then be expected to carry out this task.

In addition to clearing and preparing the work area after a treatment, the salon furnishings and equipment should be kept clean at all times. The best way to make sure that everything is cleaned regularly is to write a list of all the cleaning jobs that need doing. There will be some jobs that need doing everyday, and others that are required only once a week. If a salon has an 'end-of-day' and a 'weekly' cleaning list, these jobs can be ticked off and signed each time they are done.

The salon supervisor and employees can then easily check to see what cleaning jobs still need doing.

Daily cleaning job	Date and therapist signature				
	25/11	26/11	27/11	28/11	29/11
Clean wax pot	SJ				
Sweep floor	SJ				
Wipe down work surfaces and trolleys	JD				
Change couch roll on trolleys	LL				
Sanitise, sterilise and put away tools	LL				
Clear away all equipment	LL				
Lay out fresh towels	JD				
Clean mirrors	SJ				

An example of a daily cleaning list for a treatment room

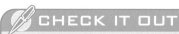

CHECK IT OUT

Think about the salon where you are learning or carrying out your work experience. Create a table with two columns – **End-of-day cleaning** and **Weekly cleaning**. Write down as many cleaning jobs as you can think of.

When you have finished, compare your list with other students in the class.

Hot and cold running water

The salon must have a constant supply of hot and cold running water. Each treatment room should have a separate sink with hot and cold running water. However, if a large treatment room has been separated into treatment bays by curtains, then a central sink will do.

The water supply is used for sanitising hands and tools, cleaning the room, and parts of the treatment, for example, mask removal.

Your responsibilities at work: working with water

Report to your supervisor *immediately*:

- blocked sinks, so that they don't overflow
- water that comes out of the tap a funny colour
- any leak, loose tap or cracked pipe.

INFORMATION

Dirty water smells unpleasant and encourages the growth of bacteria, which can cause illness.

Don't:

■ leave taps running, especially the hot water tap as this is wasteful and very expensive for the salon

■ flush mask products or other semi-solid products down the sink

■ tip chemicals, solvents or cleaning agents down the treatment room sink.

Lighting

Lighting gives a salon atmosphere, so the wrong lighting can have a disastrous effect on how the client feels when she walks in to the reception, her level of relaxation once in the treatment room, and whether she feels as though she has had a satisfying treatment at the end.

In reception

The lighting needs to be bright enough in reception so that:

■ products for sale are shown clearly

■ appointment systems are easy to read

■ manicures can be carried out.

A good overhead light and windows that allow ample daylight into the room are ideal.

In the treatment room

The lighting in the treatment rooms should be:

■ bright enough to carry out treatments and;

■ soft enough to enable clients to relax.

Therefore it is recommended that a treatment room has a good overhead light on a dimmer switch, and a magnifying lamp for close work such as skin inspection.

Safety

Make sure that:

■ you can always see clearly

■ you and your client don't squint because lighting is poor, or become dazzled by lights that are too bright

■ you always report flickering or faulty lights to your supervisor.

The treatment room

The treatment room is used for a variety of different treatments. It is therefore important that it can be adapted to meet the needs of a range of treatments and is well equipped.

The treatment room should:

■ be well ventilated – cool in summer, warm in winter

■ be quiet and undisturbed from outside noise; soft music can be played to enhance relaxation

■ have good lighting that can be dimmed for massage

- be clean, tidy and fresh smelling
- contain everything you need for treatments, and be well organised
- not be cramped, with enough space for the beauty therapist to walk round the room easily
- contain shelves or storage for products and towels
- have a sink with running hot and cold water
- include somewhere to hang the client's clothes.

INFORMATION

One of your responsibilities will be to set up the treatment room or area for the therapist.
- Setting up for a facial and manicure is covered in Section 4 (pages 94 and 131). This section also includes information on the essential tools and equipment needed.
- When setting up for waxing, make-up, eye treatments or pedicures, the only real difference is that the products change.

Things that you need to prepare the treatment room

You will need to collect the client record card from reception and check what treatment the client is booked in for, so that you know what you need to set up. (Manicure and facial requirements are covered fully in Section 4, pages 100–7 and 138–44.)

 REMEMBER

Each workplace has its own methods for setting up so use the table on page 36 as a guide.

A place to relax and unwind

An employer has a duty to provide space in which employees can rest and eat. A staff room or separate area is important because it is not acceptable to eat in the reception or treatment areas. Even drinks in the salon should be reserved for clients, in order to maintain a professional image.

The staff room should have an area for staff coats and preferably lockers for valuables, for example, handbags and expensive beauty therapy tools. A separate toilet and washing facility would also be ideal, however, this is not always possible and staff may have to share the toilet with clients. If this is the case, staff must give their clients *preference* and make sure that they leave the room spotless at all times.

First choice.

A staff area with comfortable seating, tea- and coffee-making facilities and a microwave oven would also benefit the wellbeing of staff.

In the beauty industry, you are there to provide a service to clients, so there is not much time to relax and unwind. If you work in a successful salon, you will be rushed off your feet. Don't be under the illusion that it's an easy job!

	Basics	Tech tools	Lotions and potions
Waxing	Record card Wax pot containing enough wax Dry cotton wool Wax strips Plastic sheet on couch Protective tissue for couch and client Modesty towel Two waste bins with liners (one for wax waste, the other for general waste) Sterilising jar for scissors and tweezers Disposable gloves After-care leaflet	Disposable spatulas Disposable orange sticks Tweezers Scissors	Pre-wax cleaner Talcum powder After-wax lotion
Eye treatments These include: Eyelash tinting Eyebrow tinting Eyebrow shaping	Record card Hand mirror Damp cotton wool squares Half moons for eyelash tinting Bowl of clean water Protective tissue for client and couch Towel Waste bin Sterilising jar for tweezers Tissues Disposable gloves	Disposable eyelash brush Eyebrow brush Two covered orange sticks Sterilised tweezers	Eyelash tint 2 per cent peroxide Vaseline Antiseptic solution After-care lotion
Make-up	Record card Hand mirror Damp cotton wool squares Dry cotton wool Protective tissue for client and couch Protective gown or cape Towel Headband Tissues	Clean, sterilised make-up brushes Palette	Full range of make-up Cleanser Toner Moisturiser
Manicure and Facial treatments	See appropriate chapters.		
Pedicure	The same as for the manicure plus a foot spa with hot soapy water and disposable toe separators.		

Setting-up procedure for treatments

Fresh air

Ventilation is needed to ensure a good circulation of fresh air in the salon. It is also important that the rooms are warm enough for the clients to undress for treatments.

The means for bringing fresh air into a room.

What happens when there is a lack of fresh air?

▪ Illnesses spread because of germs and bacteria circulating around the salon.

▪ A smelly and stuffy atmosphere is created, which is unpleasant for staff and clients.

▪ There is a build-up of fumes from glues, varnish and cleaning products, which can cause headaches and sickness.

Methods of ventilation

▪ Extractor fans.

▪ Windows.

▪ Air vents.

▪ Doors.

▪ *flues*.

The ideal temperature

The HSE states that in beauty therapy:

▪ the ideal working temperature is between 15.5 and 20.0 degrees Celsius

▪ the level of moisture in the air should be between 30 and 70 per cent.

A pipe through which hot air is removed from a building.

In salons and spas that have steam and sauna areas, it is important that the air does not become too damp and humid, so good ventilation is essential.

There are many different heating methods, however, many are either too expensive to run on a regular basis, or are not good enough at heating large areas. Therefore, the best method of heating is **thermostatically controlled gas central heating**. Thermostatically controlled heating can easily be turned up or down, and every room is fitted with a radiator. When it is installed by a qualified engineer and checked annually, it is the best and most cost effective way to heat a salon.

Insurance

What you will learn about:

In this section, you will learn about the types of insurance that are needed at work:

▪ Employer's Liability (Compulsory Insurance) Act 1969

▪ Professional Indemnity Insurance

▪ Buildings Insurance

▪ Contents Insurance

Employer's Liability Insurance

You must have it.

This insurance is **compulsory** for employers and business owners. All employees, clients and visitors to the salon must be covered under this insurance in case they injure themselves or catch a disease at work. The Certificate of Insurance must be displayed in the workplace for all to see. It will include the following details:

- the name of the business and owner
- the type of business
- the start date and end date of the insurance
- the name of the insurance company.

EverSure PLC

"CERTIFICATE OF EMPLOYERS' LIABILITY INSURANCE (A)

(Where required by regulation 5 of the Employers' Liability (Compulsory Insurance) Regulations 1998 (the Regulations), one or more copies of this certificate must be displayed in each place of business at which the policy holder employs persons covered by the policy)

	Policy No	R3/21LG52123
	Reference No	92L31
1.	Name of policy holder.	Mrs Tiffany Tsang trading as Top Tips
2.	Date of commencement of insurance policy.	31 July 2004
3.	Date of expiry of insurance.	31 July 2005

We hereby certify that subject to paragraph 2:–

1.   the policy to which this certificate relates satisfies the requirements of the relevant law applicable in Great Britain, Northern Ireland, the Isle of Man, the Island of Jersey, the Island of Guernsey and the Island of Alderney (b); and

2   (a)   the minimum amount of cover provided by this policy is no less than £5 million (c).

Signed on behalf of EverSure plc (Authorised Insurer)

R J Stanley

R J Stanley
CHIEF EXECUTIVE OFFICER UK

Notes

(a) Where the employer is a company to which regulation 3(2) of the Regulations applies, the certificate shall state in a prominent place, either that the policy covers the holding company and all its subsidiaries, or that the policy covers the holding company and all its subsidiaries except any specially excluded by name, or that the policy covers the holding company and only the name subsidiaries.

(b) Specify applicable law as provided for in regulation 4(5) of the Regulations.

(c) See regulation 3(1) of the Regulations and delete whichever of paragraphs 2(a) or 2(b) does not apply. Where 2(b) is applicable, specify the amount of cover provided by the relevant policy."

paragraph 2(b) does not apply and is deleted.

fold -- fold

YOUR CERTIFICATE OF EMPLOYERS' LIABILITY INSURANCE IS ATTACHED ABOVE.

THE EMPLOYERS' LIABILITY (COMPULSORY INSURANCE) REGULATIONS 1998 REQUIRE YOU TO KEEP THIS CERTIFICATE OR A COPY FOR 40 YEARS.

Please fold as shown and insert the certificate in the protective cover provided. A copy of the certificate must be displayed at all places where you employ persons covered by the policy. Extra copies of the certificate are available on request.

An Employer's Liability Insurance Certificate

Professional Indemnity Insurance

This insurance covers claims against employees if they cause injury or damage to a client or client's property through their irresponsible actions and behaviour. If an employee doesn't take out this insurance, then they must make sure that they are fully covered on the Employer's Liability Insurance.

Building Insurance

If the salon building is rented or leased from a property owner, then he or she will be responsible for insuring it against fire or damage. However, if the building is owned by the salon, then the owner will need to take out this Building Insurance.

Contents Insurance

In addition, the contents of the business will need to be insured against accidental damage, fire or theft. Contents Insurance covers items such as:

- tools and equipment
- products
- furniture
- valuables.

Carelessness and lack of attention.

This insurance will not cover damage caused through **negligence** or by natural wear and tear.

Security and safekeeping

What you will learn about:

In this section, you will learn about how to protect the workplace, clients and products from theft. You will cover:

- the salon
- staff and clients
- stock.

The salon

A salon owner needs to make sure that the business premises are secure. The salon will not be covered on insurance for fire, theft or damage if it is not. It is therefore vital that the correct steps are carried out to secure the building.

■ **When closed:**

- All external doors must be locked when the building is empty.
- All windows must be shut and locked at the end of the day.
- Burglar alarms must be turned on.
- All money must be banked daily and not left on the premises or in the till.
- The till must be emptied at the end of the day and left open.
- A security nightlight should be installed, to deter burglars.
- A trustworthy person, either a member of staff or a neighbour, should be given a spare key in case of emergency; the person's name and address should be given to the police.

■ **When open:**

- Senior members of staff should bank money regularly.
- There should be a secure safe for money that cannot be banked until later in the day.
- There should be an electronic till which is used by one or two members of staff only.
- All visitors must be checked in at reception.

Health and Safety at Work Act 1974

Within this Act it states that all employers must provide a safe system of **cash handling**. For example, if an employee is sent to the bank to pay money in alone and is then robbed or mugged, the employer could be prosecuted.

 REMEMBER

As a trainee, it is not your responsibility to take money to the bank for paying in or to handle large amounts of money.

Staff and clients

To avoid loss, theft or damage of goods and valuables that belong to staff and clients:

- lockers should be provided for staff valuables and handbags
- staff should avoid bringing valuables or large sums of money to work
- clients should keep their handbags and valuables with them at all times, unless client lockers are available in the salon
- clients should themselves place jewellery or valuables in their handbag, or keep such items in full view during a treatment.

Stock

To protect stock against theft:

- the stock cupboard should remain locked and the key kept in a safe place, preferably in the office
- one or two senior members of staff should be responsible for giving out stock for treatments and refilling of products
- products for retail should be kept in full view of the reception desk in a locked display cabinet. The key for the cabinet should be placed on a hook behind the reception desk, where it cannot be seen or reached by visitors
- if a locked cabinet is not available for displaying products, the empty boxes should be put on display and the products kept in the locked stock cupboard
- carry out weekly stock checks to make sure that the amounts of stock match with what *should* be there.

Highlight on health and safety

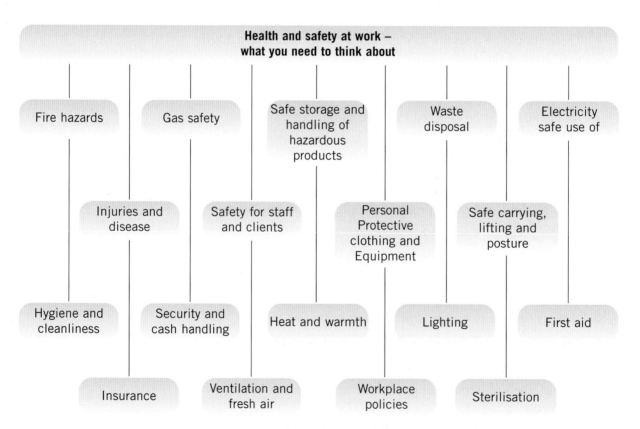

Health and Safety – what you need to think about

SALON STORY

Eve welcomed her client into the treatment room. She took her coat and excess clothing and asked her to get onto the couch. Next, Eve explained that she was going to wash her hands and collect her tools from the steriliser.

Eve collected her tools and placed them in the pocket of her uniform so that she could carry the towels. A pair of tweezers fell out of her pocket and, as she bent to pick them up, she dropped the towels. Eve picked up the tweezers and placed them in the disinfectant solution and then collected some fresh clean towels from the cupboard and placed the dropped ones in the laundry basket.

Eve prepared the client for an eye treatment by cleansing off the make-up from around the eyes. She explained that the therapist would be along shortly to continue with her treatment. Suddenly, Eve sneezed. She managed to turn away from the client in time to put her hand in front of her mouth. 'Bless you,' said the client, and handed Eve a tissue from her pocket. Eve thanked the client, placed the tissue in the waste bin and continued with the final cleansing around the eyes.

Read through the passage. What did Eve do right, and what did she do wrong? List the points and your reasons for them.

 MEMORY JOGGER

1 What are workplace policies?

2 What are the three ways of keeping the salon and equipment clean and hygienic?

3 What are your responsibilities in the workplace for safety regarding:
   - fire
   - electricity
   - hygiene?

4 What is a risk assessment?

5 What is a risk and what is a hazard? Give two examples of each.

6 Why is it important to maintain high standards of hygiene?

7 What is cross-infection? How can it be prevented?

8 What insurance *must* a salon have? What other insurance *might* a salon have?

9 List as many ways as you can for making the salon secure.

Introduction

In this unit, you will learn about the qualities needed as a beauty therapy receptionist. It is a very important job. If reception duties are not carried out properly, this could result in confusion, a loss of bookings, a drop in takings, and a bad name for the salon. As salon receptionist, the success of the salon - how busy it is and the reputation it has - could depend on you! This may sound drastic, however, you should remember that nearly all clients decide whether they like or dislike a salon within the first ten seconds of entering.

The role of salon receptionist is very demanding. Could you be enthusiastic, bright and cheerful, helpful, *professional* and *respectful* to every client that walks through the salon doors, whatever mood you're in? If not, then this chapter will help you to improve your *techniques* for dealing with clients.

Acting according to high working standards and a good attitude.

Treating others with politeness and thought.

Practical skills.

■ You will focus on how you communicate with clients, work colleagues and your manager.

■ You will also look at the personality and talent necessary to be a good receptionist – it can be easy to assume that you are doing a good job, without recognising the skills that are actually required.

Occasionally a salon will employ an experienced receptionist who is not a beauty therapist. However, it is more usual for existing beauty staff to take turns in running the reception. This approach is probably best because beauty staff have a good knowledge of the different treatments, and can therefore give better advice and guidance to clients without the need for extra training.

Reception duties allow beauty staff to gain 'hands-on' experience in:

■ making appointments

■ attending to clients

- selling products

- money handling

- communication

- numeracy skills, for example, counting money, giving correct change, taking money for sales and treatments, and stocktaking

- the different working pressures experienced by both a receptionist and a beauty therapist.

In this unit, you will cover the following topics:

- you, the receptionist

- the smooth running of reception

- attending to clients and enquiries

- helping to make appointments.

You, the receptionist

What you will learn about:
- Personal presentation
- How to welcome clients
- A professional attitude
- Working together
- Understanding each other

Personal presentation

It is essential that the receptionist's appearance is of a very high standard. Most clients will think that the way the receptionist appears reflects the standards in the salon. So, if the staff are sloppy and untidy in appearance, then a client may think that the staff are not skilled at carrying out beauty treatments.

Appearance: a checklist for success

- Wear smart clothes or uniform – they should be freshly laundered and not smell of smoke or strong perfumes.
- Your uniform or clothes should not be too short or too tight, and must allow for easy movement while carrying out treatments.
- Your hair should be clean and neat.
- Wear light, but attractive, day make-up; definitely not heavy make-up.
- Your nails should be neatly manicured – no chipped nail varnish.
- Keep your breath fresh – no tobacco smells.
- If you wear jewellery, it should be simple and kept to a minimum.

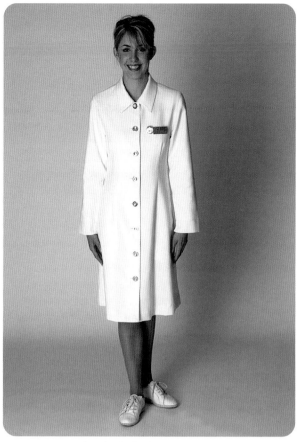
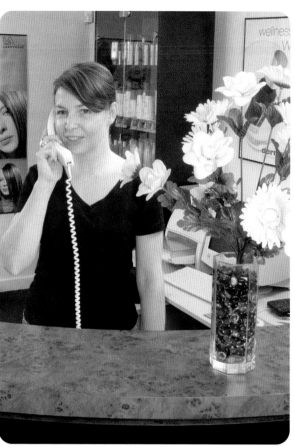

It is important that both the beauty therapist and the receptionist look smart

How to welcome clients

The value of a warm welcome for clients must not be underestimated – a warm and bright smile that is genuine will instantly put a client at ease.

Welcoming clients: a checklist for success

- Make eye contact without staring and keep your facial expressions open – don't frown, roll your eyes or glare.
- Don't chat to other members of staff while a client is with you, unless it is to answer an enquiry about their appointment or treatment. Remember to keep information *confidential*.
- Vary the tone of your voice so that you don't sound bored and disinterested. Ask helpful questions to show interest in your client.
- Be caring and *discreet*. Remember – many clients feel quite nervous about visiting a beauty salon.

Keeping things that a client tells you private.

Careful in your choice of words and able to keep secrets.

A professional attitude

If you want to be part of the Beauty Industry, you need to show many positive qualities. Sometimes it is not easy to act positively, especially if you are not feeling great – you may have had a sleepless night or a row with a friend. However, there can be *no* excuses for anything less than a professional attitude. As a beauty salon receptionist, you are on show to every client that visits the salon. You must therefore be able to carry out your duties to a high standard, no matter how you feel.

REMEMBER

As a beauty therapist, your job is to make your clients feel more relaxed and better about themselves.

SALON STORY

Sunita rushed into the salon, ten minutes late. Her bus had failed to arrive on time again!

It was Sunita's turn on reception today, and she hated it. She walked past two clients who were already waiting and dumped her handbag on the desk. Then she took out her make-up bag. She wanted to put her make-up on before her boss saw her. She was glad that no one caught her doing this. She eyed one of the women in the waiting area who was huffing and tutting. Sunita became annoyed. She always seemed to get lumbered with the awkward clients.

Janie, the head therapist, came into reception. She went straight to Sunita and told her off for not letting her know that her client had arrived. Sunita rolled her eyes – it was going to be one of those days. The phone rang. Sunita lifted the receiver but replaced it straight away, as she was not yet organised. She still needed to change into her uniform, put her bag in her locker and make a coffee to wake herself up.

Sunita went through to the staff room, where she chatted and giggled for a few minutes about the party she went to last night. Then she sorted herself out.

Sunita 's day soon went from bad to worse. The salon manager called her into her office and gave her a verbal warning about her conduct and attitude. She said that she was responsible for therapists starting treatments late, make-up on the appointment sheets and a theft in reception. To Sunita, this was terribly unfair. She was always the person that was blamed when anything went wrong. She decided that she would start looking for another job.

1 List the things that Sunita did wrong.

2 Comment on her attitude. Was it acceptable?

3 How could Sunita improve her morning routine and make herself a more popular staff member?

Working together

Working with other people in a salon is not always easy. It can be necessary for very different personalities to work together in a small environment. Being helpful and supportive while making a *positive contribution* to the team effort will help you to achieve success with both your workmates and your manager.

Give helpful ideas and work hard.

REMEMBER

A successful business employs reliable and hard-working staff who work well together as a team.

Unfortunately, you won't always have great relationships with your colleagues at work. You will need to accept that everyone you work with is different. You are not expected to like all your colleagues, however, you must be able to get along with them. This means that you must respect each other's differences and build good working relationships.

To work successfully as part of a team, you need to listen to other people's views even though you may not agree with them. When you want to put an important point across, you should speak in a calm voice without showing *aggression*. There is more chance that you will be taken seriously and listened to if you don't get angry or lose your temper. Making *tactless remarks* could hurt or offend people. Remember, there is always room for different views and opinions.

Anger, annoyance or loss of temper.

Remarks made without any thought or consideration as to how they will annoy or upset the person who hears them.

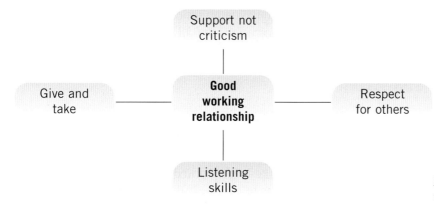

Factors contributing to good working relationships

Teamwork

Teamwork is also about give and take. There are always jobs to do which are less popular than others, or times when staff are needed to do *overtime.* Don't let it always be the same people who put in the extra effort. If that person is always you, you should be prepared to say 'no' and suggest a fairer system. If you always sneak off when jobs need doing, ask yourself, 'Am I being fair?'

Extra hours that you work on top of your set hours.

 REMEMBER

As a beauty therapist, you should aim to be hard working and reliable. This means that you work to the best of your abilities and don't need constant supervision. Flexibility is also a great advantage. Try to *adapt* to changing circumstances and situations without complaining.

Change in order to meet different needs.

You need to have a lot of respect for your colleagues to ensure good staff relations. Problems that occur should be talked about immediately. If they are not talked about, **resentment** will build up and this will lead to a strained atmosphere. This negative atmosphere may be picked up by clients and other staff members, affecting the salon as a whole.

Dislike, bitterness or anger.

CHECK IT OUT

This task is designed as a group discussion, so that you use **teamwork** to benefit from other people's ideas.

Describe the 'ideal' working colleague using a spidergram (there is an example of a spidergram on page 47).

Understanding each other

INFORMATION

The key to all good relationships, whether personal, business or work relationships, is effective communication. There are many different forms of communication, but all are built on our ability to pass on information, feelings and understanding through speaking, writing or body language.

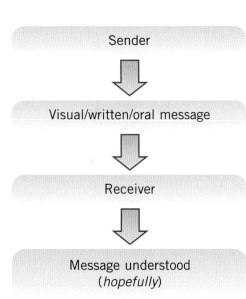

Sender

↓

Visual/written/oral message

↓

Receiver

↓

Message understood
(*hopefully*)

↓

Feedback/reply given

A flow chart to show the process of communication

Communication is a two-way process. Its success depends on how clearly we can make ourselves understood, and how clearly we can understand others. We usually take it for granted that we have made ourselves clear to others. If there's a communication problem, it's easy to think that it's the other person's fault and not ours. However, even when writing the words on this page, I can't be completely sure that you understand me, all I can do is try to make my words as clear as possible.

Methods of communication

- **Verbal** – speaking to another person. This includes speaking by telephone or face-to-face conversations.
- **Non-verbal** – eye contact, body language or sign language, not spoken language.
- **Visual** – pictures that communicate information, for example, in adverts, posters, magazines and brochures.
- **Written** – for example, in letters, memos, faxes, text messages and email.

CHECK IT OUT

Below is a list of some of the different tasks that a receptionist must perform. Your task is to match the correct method of communication to each task. Some of the methods are quicker than others are, so you will need to prioritise. In other words, decide how important or urgent the message is, then decide on the best method of communication.

You may like to copy the chart below then draw a line to connect each task with the correct method.

Task	Method of communication
To let a therapist know that her next client has cancelled an appointment	Invoice
To inform all staff of the extended opening times in the salon	Meeting
To let all staff know about the new arrangements in the staff room	Memo
To tell customers about new products	Noticeboard
To inform a client how much she owes	Poster
To discuss the staff performance and pay rise	Spoken word

CHECK IT OUT

How do we know if our method of communication has worked?

In pairs, discuss how we can tell if our message has been understood.

Your style of communication

In the Beauty Industry, you will need to communicate with clients when giving *client consultations*, advice and aftercare, and when selling products and treatments. You will also need to build good relationships with clients and pass on important information. You therefore need to make sure not only that you speak clearly, but also that your **style** of communicating is appropriate.

Question and answer sessions with a client that are designed to find out information about them.

- **Positive methods:**
  - Talking calmly and quietly.
  - Smiling.
  - Touching.
  - Using approachable body language, for example, arms unfolded, legs uncrossed, facing a client and not turning your back.
  - Eye contact.
  - Simple language that a client understands easily.
  - Open, welcoming gestures such as shaking hands to welcome a client.
  - Maintaining good posture.

■ **Negative methods:**

■ Shouting.

■ Gossiping.

■ Showing negative reactions, for example, by sneering, rolling the eyes or tutting.

■ Showing impatience or boredom, for example, by sighing or yawning.

■ Making too much eye contact – a client might think that you're staring and feel uneasy.

Informal language and speech

■ Using *slang*, for example, 'hiya', 'see ya', 'hang on a minute'.

■ Texting and making private phone calls.

■ Showing bad posture, for example, slouching, leaning on your hands, putting your hands on your hips or in your pockets.

These negative methods are all **barriers to communication** and should never be used at work.

 CHECK IT OUT

Divide the positive and negative methods of communication into verbal and non-verbal methods.

When you have finished, add more examples of positive and negative communication to the list.

 SALON STORY

It was a very busy Saturday morning in the salon. The reception was buzzing with clients waiting for treatments and buying products. Debbie noticed a woman hovering outside the door looking very unsure of herself. She wondered whether the woman wanted to see a brochure or book a treatment, or whether she was just waiting for someone. Debbie wasn't sure what she should say to her.

Then Lisa, the salon junior, called to the woman over the heads of the other clients, saying 'Come in, we don't bite!' The woman came in rather sheepishly. Debbie asked. 'How can we help?' The woman explained in a whispered voice that she was interested in waxing. 'What part of the body?' called out Lisa from the other end of the desk. The woman winced. She didn't want to say in front of all the other people, so took a brochure and hurried out saying that she would telephone later.

❶ Could this matter have been dealt with better? How?

❷ Was the communication between the woman and staff good? Why?

❸ Do you think that the woman will return to the salon? Give a reason for your answer.

The smooth running of reception

What you will learn about:

▪ The purpose of a reception area

▪ The importance of the reception surroundings

▪ The organisation of stationery and paperwork

▪ Confidential information and the Data Protection Act

▪ Product displays and stock

The purpose of a reception area

Perhaps the key purpose of the reception area is the booking of appointments, both on the telephone and in person. There are, however, many more reasons why a beauty salon needs a reception.

▪ It is the first point of contact for clients.

▪ It is where information and help on treatments and products are provided.

▪ It is where the sale of products and the handling of money for product sales and treatments takes place.

▪ It is used for handing out brochures and pricelists to *potential clients*.

▪ Window and cabinet display for products, and possibly even flower displays, will be set up here.

▪ It is where appointments are booked and enquiries are dealt with by telephone and in person.

▪ It is where clients are looked after, both before and after treatment.

People who are interested in beauty treatments and may use the salon in the future.

The importance of the reception surroundings
The reception area from outside

For people in the street – who may be potential clients – the reception area is an extension of the shop window. As they look into the salon, they will see the reception area. It is therefore important that the reception area appears organised and very clean, and gives a *good impression* of the salon.

The *shop front* should encourage clients to enter, so it must have:

▪ plants or hanging baskets

▪ information about the salon's hours of opening

▪ signs saying what treatments are available

▪ clean windows

▪ a freshly painted exterior – not cracked or peeling

▪ a well-swept front.

When you have a positive feeling or opinion about someone or something.

The outside of the salon.

However, while it is good to have a central position in a busy shopping area for a beauty salon, it is best not to be in full view of passing people. Blinds can therefore be used to screen waiting clients from public view, and to shade display products from a hot sun.

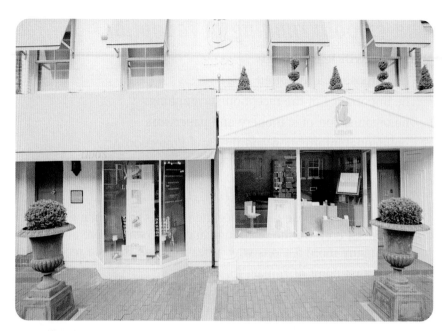

The outside of the beauty salon should encourage people to want to enter

Inside the reception area

When a client enters the reception area, he or she needs to feel welcome and at ease with the staff and surroundings. It is also important that clients have the impression that the salon is being run professionally and efficiently.

The whole reception area should be well lit, warm, fresh smelling and, most importantly, spotless. There should be a comfortable seating area for waiting clients with a selection of up-to-date magazines and promotion leaflets. The temperature should be warm in the cooler seasons, and airy in the summer months. Refreshments in the form of tea, coffee and mineral water should be available for clients, both before and after treatment. Relaxing background music should be played to create a relaxed atmosphere and enhance clients' experience of the salon.

In the reception area, there should be a locked product display cabinet from which a client can view and purchase skin, body and nail care products. All salon staff should be familiar with the products so that they can advise clients. If you notice that stocks are low, inform the correct staff member.

The general decoration of a room.

The **décor** of the salon should reflect the image that the salon wants to achieve. The colours and textures of the walls, ceilings, furniture, linen and towels should work together to create the correct atmosphere of tranquillity and relaxation. A more modern and funky approach to design is not recommended, as it can date very quickly. It is best to aim for a classic design, using pale colours for a fresh look.

The organisation of stationery and paperwork

The reception desk should be positioned so that the receptionist can greet all people that enter the salon. It should be neat and tidy at all times with just the essentials on view – the cash till, the appointment

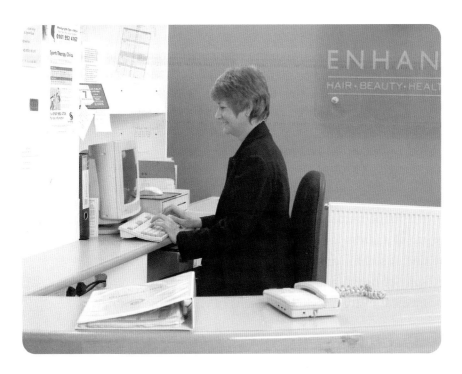

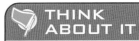

The salon reception desk should be neat and tidy at all times

book, price lists, appointment cards, the telephone, and a pencil, eraser and pen.

Ideally, the reception desk should have shelving underneath the desk. This allows for larger amounts of stationery and paperwork to be stored in an orderly way without cluttering up the desk. It also makes it easy to see at a glance when brochures, appointment cards and appointment sheets are getting low and need to be reordered.

> **REMEMBER**
>
> If you notice that salon stationery is getting low, take responsibility and inform the member of staff who deals with stock and ordering.

Confidential information and the Data Protection Act
Record systems

Confidential information, such as client records, should never be visible to other clients or to members of staff not treating the client. They should be stored in drawers underneath the reception desk.

While on reception duty, you will see clients' private records. You have *no* right to pass these on or to talk about them to anyone, except other members of staff who need to know because they may carry out a treatment on or look after the client. Even then, you must only discuss client details when it concerns a work-related matter and you have the permission of the client. If you are unsure about what to do, ask a senior member of staff.

> **THINK ABOUT IT**
>
> What beauty salons are there in your area? Have you visited them? If you have, think about their reception area, what they do right and what they could improve on. Discuss in pairs or as a group.

Keeping all personal information that a client tells you private.

Confidential information

Confidentiality is central to the running of a professional beauty salon. A client must feel confident that any personal information she gives remains private, and that the staff don't gossip about her behind her back. Gossiping about clients is unprofessional behaviour that breaks a client's trust and is extremely disrespectful to the client.

What information is confidential?

The client's:

* name and addresses
* telephone number
* email address
* doctor's name and address
* state of health and record of any illness
* medical history, including details of current medication.

 REMEMBER

Information is given by a client to a therapist in confidence. This information *must* remain private unless it is illegal or could hurt someone. If you are unsure or worried about confidentiality, always check with your manager.

The Data Protection Act

The Data Protection Act covers many different working practices. The section that is important to beauty therapists is the section that describes the **correct privacy methods** that should be in place in a salon. These privacy methods ensure that it is difficult for other people to get hold of, look at or use a person's private details without permission, for any reason.

The Act states that we should treat a client's personal details **in confidence** – that means keeping it private. It is against the law to give out someone's personal information without his or her permission.

INFORMATION

Never leave a record card on the reception desk in full view of everyone.

Never allow clients to view a person's record card on a computer screen.

Product displays and stock
Product on display

Skincare and cosmetics are attractive products to clients – we all love new make-up, nail varnishes and skin creams. If attractively displayed and on show to passing clients, it is likely that these products will sell easily.

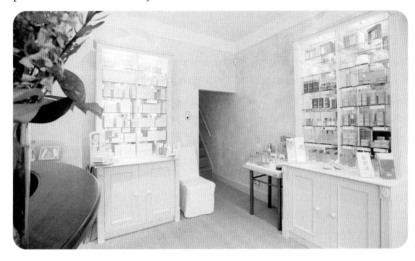

A product display

The best way to display products is in the reception area in a locked glass-fronted cabinet. The cabinet should be positioned away from the glare and direct heat of the sun. This is because:

- the sun will bleach the boxes and thicken and spoil the creams and varnishes
- the heat could cause the products to thicken and separate.

The products should be neatly arranged and clearly visible to the eye. There should be enough products on display to catch people's interest without them looking cluttered. One or two of each item that you stock is enough.

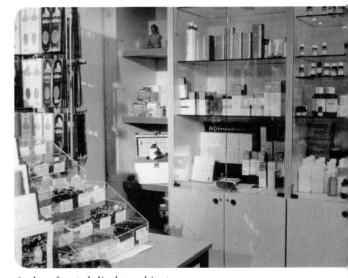

A glass-fronted display cabinet

The products should look as new as when they were first put on display. It is therefore important that they are taken out and dusted regularly. If the products are dusty or look old, it will discourage people from buying them. Any breakages or faulty products will need to be taken out of the display cabinet and reported straight away to the relevant person.

Stock storage

The main stock should be stored out of view, but in an easy-to-reach location, so that when a sale is made the product can be accessed easily. It is also good for the client to see that she is purchasing a new product and not one that has been used for display purposes.

Shelf life

Remember that all stock has a **shelf life**. This means that it has a recommended time limit during which it should be stored or used. After this time, the product can go off making it unfit for use. Outward signs that a product has gone off are:

- an unpleasant smell
- **separation** – this is when a cream or lotion is no longer completely mixed together and becomes part cream, part liquid
- **thickness** – if a product has passed its sell-by date or has been open to the air, it can turn hard where it becomes *dehydrated*
- **discoloration** – this is when a product changes colour.

Loses moisture.

Stock rotation

To ensure that products are used within their shelf life and do not go off, a system known as **stock rotation** is used.

- New stock received from suppliers is placed at the back of the storage area so that it is sold last.
- Stock already on the premises is stored at the front and is sold first.

If your salon does not sell a lot of stock, then products will be sitting in storage for some time and sell-by dates will need to be checked on a regular basis and less stock carried. A common solution when stock is reaching its sell-by date is to promote it as a special offer and sell it at a discounted price.

> ### CHECK IT OUT
>
> Think of a beauty product that you would like to sell. To ensure stock is sold before its sell-by date, you are going to advertise this product at a discounted price and design a 'special offer' poster, to be displayed in the reception area. The special offer could be a percentage or a half-price discount, or a buy-one-get-one-free offer.
>
> Remember to make the poster colourful, tasteful and easy to read. It must be eye-catching!

Correct storage of stock

To prevent spoilage and extend a product's shelf life, it should be stored as follows:

- keep dry and cool
- keep in a dark place away from sunlight
- keep away from naked flame
- keep in an airtight container – for example, if you open a face cream and then try to reseal it, it will be unfit for sale.

However, you should always check the manufacturer's instructions about correct product storage.

Recording stock levels

Stock should be checked in and out of the salon using either a notebook (the *manual* method) or a computer (a computerised system). If stock levels are not recorded properly, it is impossible to know when to reorder products and which ones to reorder. It is also impossible to check which products are popular with clients, and whether any have been stolen.

By hand.

When stock is counted on a regular basis, this is called a **stocktake**.

Stocktaking

- When carrying out a stocktake, there should be a list of available stock for sale and salon use either in a file, notebook or on the computer.
- All staff should record when a new product is opened for use in the salon, and when an old product is empty and the bottle or tub is discarded.
- All sales and breakages should be recorded.
- Ideally, a stocktake should be done each week, so that available stock is counted and a list made of new stock to be ordered.
- A stocktake is best done using a **stock sheet**.

Using a stock sheet

When new stock arrives in the salon, each individual item needs to be entered into the amount column. It is not advisable to enter the total amount of stock in one cell, as this would make it difficult to count out. For example, if you receive four cleansers, you should mark '1' in the amount column four times. In this way, stock can easily be checked out by crossing through each '1'.

Once you have entered the product and the amount of stock, then you can complete the column for 'Date in'. When stock is removed from the stock cupboard, you should complete the columns for 'Date

Product	Date in	Amount	Date out	Reason	Signature
Cleanser for dry skin	20/07/03	11𝟷	28/07/03	sale	SJT
		111𝟷𝟷			
		11			
		1			
Toner for dry skin	20/07/03	1	01/08/03	damaged – reported	LL
		1			

An example of a stock sheet

out' and 'Reason'. The reasons for stock being taken from the stock cupboard include:

- sale
- display
- salon use
- the stock is damaged or broken.

Finally, the person who has removed the stock must sign in the 'Signature' column. When more stock that is new arrives, enter it in the space at the bottom of the chart with the date, so it is obvious which entries are new and which are old stock.

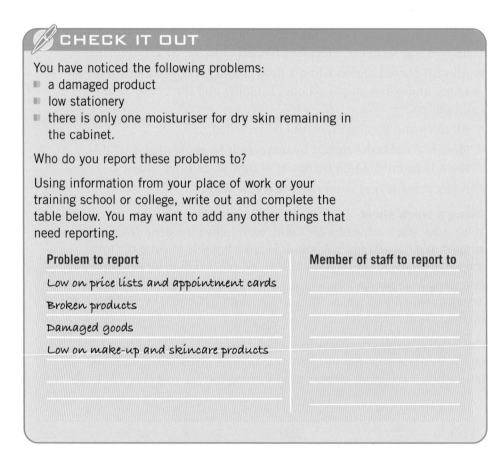

CHECK IT OUT

You have noticed the following problems:
- a damaged product
- low stationery
- there is only one moisturiser for dry skin remaining in the cabinet.

Who do you report these problems to?

Using information from your place of work or your training school or college, write out and complete the table below. You may want to add any other things that need reporting.

Problem to report	Member of staff to report to
Low on price lists and appointment cards	
Broken products	
Damaged goods	
Low on make-up and skincare products	

Attending to clients and enquiries

What you will learn about:
- Answering the telephone
- Tips for greeting clients
- Giving information and helping with sales and advice
- Taking messages
- Dealing with complaints

Answering the telephone

When chatting on the telephone to friends or family, it doesn't matter if you use slang and don't pronounce words properly. However, this is bad practice when you talk to people at work, especially when answering the telephone.

When answering the telephone at work you should:

- speak clearly, using good communication skills (as covered in the earlier section, see page 49)
- smile – even though the other person can't see you, you will sound friendlier.

The most acceptable method of telephone greeting is to use a polite greeting firstly, add the name of the salon, and then ask how you can help. Each salon usually has a preferred method of greeting when answering the telephone, and they will train their staff in this. However, the example given below is generally considered acceptable, polite and respectful without being too *formal*.

Being so careful to speak or act in the correct way that you are not very relaxed.

Tips for greeting clients

When greeting clients in person as they enter the salon, you need to speak in much the same way as when greeting clients on the telephone.

- A professional yet welcoming greeting would be:

  'Good morning/afternoon Ms/Mrs/Miss/Mr ...' (use the client's name if you know it). 'How can I be of help?'

- A professional goodbye would be:

  'We hope to see you again soon. Goodbye Ms/Mrs/Miss/Mr ...' (while holding the door open for the person).

1.Good morning/ Good afternoon

3. How can I help?

2. The Green Retreat

Telephone greeting spiral

Know your limits

When dealing with clients' appointments, enquiries and requests, it is essential that you keep within the limits of your *authority*. There will be many times when you need to pass an enquiry or request on to a senior member of staff. For example:

The limits of your power – what you are allowed to do.

- A client wishes to make an appointment and a senior staff member is busy. You don't have the authority to make the appointment. You should ask the client to take a seat and explain that you need help as you are learning. If you feel confident enough to make the booking, explain to the client that you will need to get it checked afterwards.

■ One of the salon's suppliers needs to speak to the manager, but she is at lunch and won't return for ten minutes. You should offer the supplier a coffee, show him or her the list of products that the manager wrote down in the morning, and explain that the manager will confirm what is needed when she returns from lunch.

 REMEMBER

It is great to have responsibility, but you must be aware of your limits and stick to them. Mistakes will happen if you do things that you don't have the authority to do, for example, booking a course of treatments without supervision and confirmation from a senior member of staff.

Keep your clients informed

Giving a person up-to-date information so that he or she knows what is going on.

It is very rude and unprofessional to keep a client waiting without keeping her fully *informed* of what is going on. If a client realises that she will not be dealt with immediately, then she can decide whether to wait in the salon or return later. If a client isn't kept informed of this, she may become impatient and unhappy.

Giving information and helping with sales and advice

It takes time, practice and understanding to be able to advise clients on the different products for sale and the type of treatments available. As a trainee, you can expect to be asked many questions to which you will not know the answer. However, with the help of your manager and perseverance on your part, you will gradually learn what the best advice to give is.

Below are some examples of questions that a client might ask about beauty treatments and products.

Treatments
■ What are the benefits?
■ How long does the treatment last?
■ How much does it cost?
■ How long do the effects of the treatment last?

An unpleasant response, for example, redness or soreness of the skin.

■ Can I expect any *reaction* after the treatment?
■ What do you advise for aftercare and homecare?

Products for sale
■ What are the benefits?
■ How do I use it? How do I put it on?
■ What is the correct amount to apply?
■ How long does it last?
■ How much does it cost?
■ For cleansers and moisturisers what skin type am I?

REMEMBER

It is best to refer a client to a senior member of staff rather than give out incorrect information. The consequences of giving a client incorrect information could be:

- a reaction to a product
- a double booking
- an incorrect booking which then leads to an incorrect treatment
- a returned product
- a client complaint.

 CHECK IT OUT

In pairs, choose a product and learn about it for 10–15 minutes.

Now test your knowledge. One of you will be the client; the other will be the therapist.
The client asks the therapist questions about the product, for the therapist to answer.
When you have finished, swap roles and repeat this activity for a treatment.

How much did you know? Imagine having to give information about all the products and treatments that are available in a beauty salon.

Taking messages

You will frequently be asked to take messages during your time on reception. This must be done:

- *promptly*
- *accurately*
- in writing that is neat and easy to read.

On time.
Correctly, without mistakes.

Details that you will need to write are:

1. the **date and time** of the message or call
2. **who** the message was **from**
3. **who** the message is **for**
4. **what** the message was **about**
5. **how important** the message is, for example, urgent, important or no immediate hurry
6. the caller's **name**, **company name** and **contact details** (telephone number).

INFORMATION

Message pads can help to jog a person's memory. These list all the information you should write down when taking a message and can be purchased from stationery shops.

It is very important that you remember to write down all this information, because any information that is missed could result in a complete misunderstanding. *Don't rely on memory*. When the salon is busy and you have lots of other things to remember, it is easy to forget the details of the message.

How to take messages

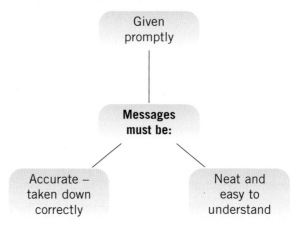

Given promptly

Messages must be:

Accurate – taken down correctly

Neat and easy to understand

CHECK IT OUT

Design your own message sheet. You may like to do this by hand or on a word processor. When you have finished, photocopy the message sheet a few times. You may like to use it when you are on reception, to see how it works!

Dealing with complaints

When a complaint is made, the reception desk is normally the first point of contact; from there, the complaint will be passed on to the appropriate senior member of staff. Since there will probably be clients waiting in reception while someone makes a complaint, it is very important that complaints are dealt with politely and without aggression. It would be embarrassing for waiting clients, and give a very poor impression of the salon, if a complaint was not handled well.

Most people dread having to deal with a complaint. Some people are very good at calming down an angry client or tackling a difficult situation. Other people react in a way that only seems to make the situation worse! What do you think that you do?

You will not be expected to sort out a complaint until much further into your training. While you are a trainee, you should pass the complaint on to the correct member of staff.

INFORMATION

Watch and learn from your workmates! You will see good and bad ways of dealing with a complaint.

Most complaints can be sorted out quickly and easily because most clients are reasonable and know exactly what will make them happy again. On the rare occasion, however, you may experience a more difficult situation that tests your patience. Whatever the situation, the client making the complaint should be gently moved away from the reception area into a quieter area of the salon, where the complaint can be dealt with privately.

> ## INFORMATION
> Be grateful. A client who complains is giving you a second chance. An unhappy client who doesn't complain will probably tell others how dissatisfied she is and never return.

Having a positive influence

When dealing with complaints, there are qualities and skills that will help solve the problem in the best way. These are:

- patience
- acting on a complaint *not* reacting
- listening skills
- deciding what are the main facts
- remaining calm
- keeping an open expression
- positive body language.

Don't forget that one of the most important and effective ways to deal with a complaint is to apologise to the client for the fact that she is unhappy with the situation. Your client could be unhappy with:

- how he or she has been treated
- the standard of treatment
- an incorrect appointment
- a faulty product that he or she purchased
- an unpleasant skin reaction to a treatment or product.

An apology will go a long way to helping your client feel better about the situation and the treatment received from the salon.

Helping to make appointments

What you will learn about:

- Booking basics
- What the client wants
- Commercially acceptable treatment timings
- When not to book an appointment

Booking basics

Salon appointments are recorded on loose sheets of paper, or in an appointment book. These contain several columns. At the top of each column, the name of the therapist is entered. The receptionist and other staff can then see clearly at a glance:

▪ which therapist is treating which client at which time

▪ which therapist has room for more appointments

▪ who is taking breaks and when.

The appointment pages are written up weeks in advance, because appointments can be made months ahead, for example, if a client is having a course of treatments. Another reason is that a client may wish to book for a special occasion such as a pre-wedding pamper, and will therefore need to book a certain date and time months in advance. Writing up the weeks ahead also helps staff to plan their holidays and work timetables can be organised around them.

Details needed when booking an appointment

1 **The client's surname.** It is not advisable to write first names because other members of staff may not know the client by their first name, nor is it a good idea to just put a surname because there may be other clients with that name. If you write the client's first initial and surname, it is easy for a therapist to look up that person's details on a record card should they need to contact the client about the booking. Another reason for using the client's surname is that some clients do not like being called by their first name.

2 **The client's telephone number.** Make sure that you write the dialling code if the telephone number is not a local number. You should also take down the client's work number if this is where the client can be contacted during working hours.

3 **The client's treatment.**

Writing in the columns

▪ Appointments must be written in **pencil only** so that mistakes or changes can be rubbed out. Don't press too hard with the pencil as it makes it hard to rub out.

▪ Your writing should be neat, clear and small. This is to allow room for all the client and treatment details to be written in a small space.

▪ It is better to print words, rather than write in a joined up style – especially if your handwriting is not very good.

THINK ABOUT IT

Imagine if a first name only was entered into the appointment book, and the incorrect telephone number was written down. How could you try to contact the client to cancel her appointment, for example, if a therapist was ill? Discuss this situation with your group and your tutor.

What the client wants

When a client contacts you to make an appointment, let her tell you exactly what she would like before interrupting her. If the client only has an idea, then help her to decide. Then repeat the information to check that you have correctly understood her wishes. If you have the authority to book the treatment, then you can do so.

We have looked at the methods for greeting clients on page 45. Now, you need to find out how to deal with the different clients who arrive in the salon.

- Clients who would like to book a treatment we will call a **New Booking**.
- Clients that are already booked and arrive for their treatment we will call an **Existing Booking**.

New booking

Steps to booking an appointment under the guidance of a senior staff member:

- Ask what treatment the client would like to book and when.
- Ask if the client would like to see a particular therapist.
- Look at the appointment book and offer some available dates and times.
- When the day, date and time have been agreed, write the client's name, telephone number and treatment in pencil only.
- Read back the day, date, time and therapist to the client to make sure that no mistakes have been made. This part is very important!
- Write down the appointment details on an appointment card to give to the client.
- Get the senior member of staff to check the entry before the client leaves.

Existing booking

- Take the client's appointment details, then get them checked by a senior staff member.
- Ask the client to take a seat in the reception area.
- Offer the client magazines and refreshments.
- Inform the therapist straight away that her next client has arrived.

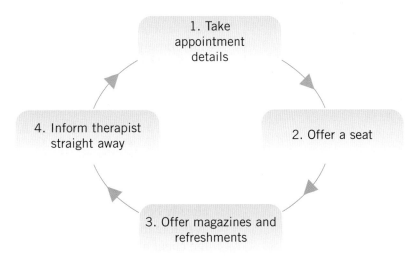

Procedure spiral for existing booking

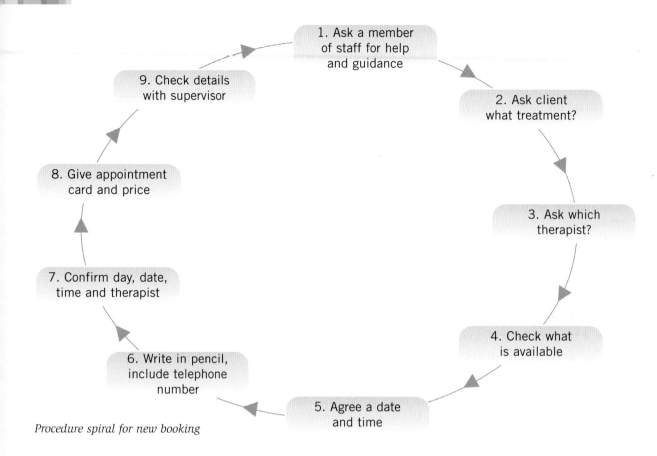

Procedure spiral for new booking

1. Ask a member of staff for help and guidance
2. Ask client what treatment?
3. Ask which therapist?
4. Check what is available
5. Agree a date and time
6. Write in pencil, include telephone number
7. Confirm day, date, time and therapist
8. Give appointment card and price
9. Check details with supervisor

THINK ABOUT IT

Two clients turn up for a treatment with the same therapist on the same day at the same time! What do you do?

INFORMATION

When making an appointment, make sure that you write in the column as you confirm the day, date and time to a client.

Never write this information in the column *after* putting the telephone down or *after* the client has left the salon. This is asking for trouble – another client could come in, the phone could ring again, a senior therapist could ask you to do some jobs for her, by which time you will have forgotten all about the appointment that you should have written down.

What to do when problems arise

- If the time that the client wants is not free, then offer the nearest time to it.
- If the client wants to see a certain therapist, but that therapist is already booked, then offer the client the next and nearest time available for that therapist. If that time is not convenient, then offer the client a different therapist.
- If an appointment needs to be changed, rub it out and rewrite it in the book and on the client's appointment card.

Commercially acceptable treatment timings
Booking out time for treatments

Another factor to think about is how long to book out for each treatment. Your manager will need to tell you how this is done for your salon, and show you how to do it. However, on nearly every appointment sheet, one line in a column stands for a 15-minute time slot. For example, if a facial takes one hour to complete, then four lines will need to be crossed through in a column.

The time taken for each treatment

There are set times for treatments and these are known as **commercially acceptable treatment times**. This is how long a treatment should take in order to make a salon money.

If you took too long to complete all your treatments, you wouldn't be able to fit many treatments into one day. You would therefore fail to make much money for the business – this would be **commercially unacceptable**.

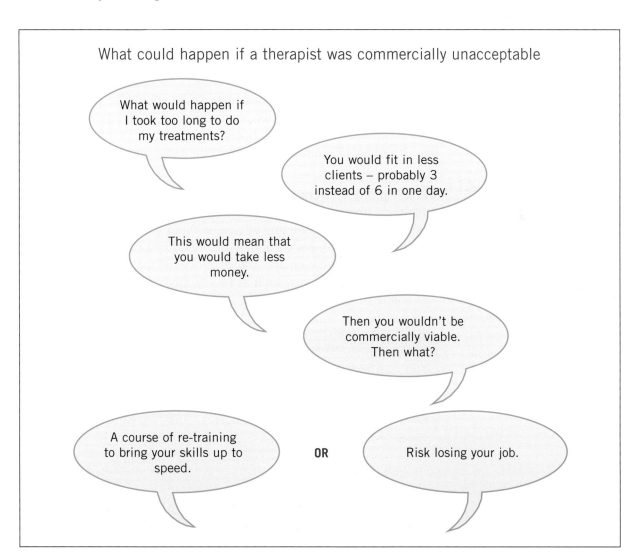

Some therapists work slightly slower or quicker than others , but still manage to complete their treatments within an acceptable time. Each therapist should let the receptionist know exactly how long she needs for each treatment.

Although it is better for a client not to be rushed out after her treatment, it is not a good idea to leave the client too long in the treatment room once the treatment has finished. This would mean that the treatment room is not available for the next client, and that the therapist is late in starting her next treatment. This delay could then have a roll-on effect for the rest of the day. By the time the last client is seen, the therapist could be an hour or so behind schedule.

To avoid the treatment room being held up in this way, the best solution is to have a relaxing area where a client can sit quietly and have a drink after her treatment. Alternatively, if the salon is large and has many treatment rooms, then it is possible that the next treatment could start in a different room while the client is left to relax where she is.

Treatment codes

As there is not much space for writing appointment details in the columns, codes are used to show which treatment has been booked. These codes vary from salon to salon, but are usually quite similar. Treatment codes are shown in the 'Code' column of the table on page 69.

When booking out some appointments, time should be allowed for client preparation, consultation, homecare and after-care advice. You should therefore book out treatment time and add 15 minutes (one line) if needed. Examples are given in the table opposite.

As a beauty therapist becomes more experienced at giving treatments, she will probably work more quickly and won't need all the time put aside for a treatment. She would therefore have extra time for preparation, consultation and advice, without the need for the receptionist to book out extra time for this. Extra time for preparation, consultation and advice is needed mainly for the larger, more relaxing treatments, such as facials, body massages and **complementary therapies**.

Treatments, such as reflexology, aromatherapy and Indian head massage, that come from alternative cultures.

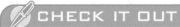

CHECK IT OUT

Write out and complete the chart on page 69 to show:
- lines to cross through
- treatment codes.

Complete this information for pedicures through to ear piercing.

Treatment	Maximum time allowed in minutes without consultation time	Preparation/ consultation time	Number of lines to cross through in appointment sheet/book	Treatment code
Eyebrow shape	15	0 – advise while treating	1	EBS
Eyelash tint	20–30	0 – advise while treating	2	ELT
Facial	60	1 – for undressing, after-care advice and tidying of work area	5	FAC
Make-up	45	0 – advise while treating	3	M-UP
Manicure	45	0 – advise while treating	3	MAN
Pedicure	45	1 – to allow drying time and putting on of shoes, also tidying of work area		
Eyebrow wax	15	0 – advise while treating		
Underarm wax	15	0 – advise while treating		
Half leg wax	30	0 – advise while treating		
Bikini wax	15	0 – advise while treating		
Arm wax	30	0 – advise while treating		
Full leg wax	45–50	0 – advise while treating		
Half leg, bikini and underarm wax	60	0 – advise while treating		
Full leg, bikini and underarm wax	75	0 – advise while treating		
Eyebrow shape and eyelash tint	30	0 – advise while treating		
Eyebrow tint	10–15	0 – advise while treating		
Eyelash tint, eyebrow tint and eyebrow shape	30	0 – advise while treating		
Ear piercing	15	0 – advise while treating		

Commercially acceptable treatment times and treatment codes

Date: **Tuesday 13th October 2003**

	Lucy	Hellena	Anetta	Siobhan	
AM 9.00	Mrs Khan	Mrs Hughes			9.00 AM
9.15	full	full			9.15
9.30	Body wax	B/Massage			9.30
9.45	01234 45678	223335			9.45
10.00					10.00
10.15					10.15
10.30		Mrs Inder			10.30
10.45	Miss Jones	Pedicure			10.45
11.00	Aroma	+ 1/2 leg wax	Miss Westerby		11.00
11.15	Back massage	01235 771540	French		11.15
11.30	357928		Manicure		11.30
11.45			+ facial		11.45
12.00			01329 815242	Mr. Vallete	12.00
12.15		Mrs Green		Back massage	12.15
12.30	LUNCH	Eye tint		+ pedicure	12.30
12.45		444321		02271 881570	12.45
PM 1.00	Mr. Walsh				1.00 PM
1.15	Manicure		Miss Rudman		1.15
1.30	+back wax	LUNCH	Miss Allen	Miss Binder	1.30
1.45	02392 815815		x2 eyebows	waxing	1.45
2.00	Mrs Suling		335215	e/b + lip & chin	2.00
2.15	Eyebrow tidy	Miss Murphy	LUNCH	07807 577211	2.15
2.30	413927	Arm wax			2.30
2.45		+ u/arm wax			2.45
3.00		223792	Miss Nair	Mrs Pattel	3.00
3.15			Bridal	Sugaring	3.15
3.30		Miss Woolford	Top to toe	to x2 leg	3.30
3.45		Basic facial +	447 812	221 335	3.45
4.00	Mrs Wang	eye lash tint			4.00
4.15	Non-surg.	445 877			4.15
4.30	facial lift				4.30
4.45	08729 815 111				4.45
5.00		Mrs Townsend			5.00
5.15		M/up			5.15
5.30		lesson			5.30
5.45		315579 ext. 222			5.45
6.00					6.00
6.15					6.15
6.30					6.30
6.45					6.45
7.00					7.00

lunchtime cover only (Siobhan column)

A page from an appointment book

When not to book an appointment

As mentioned on pages 59–60, there is a limit to your authority – the tasks you are allowed to carry out in the salon. It is important that you do not carry out activities without the permission and guidance of a senior staff member. Appointment systems can be tricky to master and easy to mess up, so ask for help where necessary. Always check appointments with a senior staff member, until you have been given permission to carry out bookings on your own.

However, there will be certain treatments or clients that you will *never* be allowed to book. Examples of these are given in the table below. Always pass these cases on to a senior member of staff.

When not to book a client	Reason why
A course of treatments	This needs careful thought and planning by the therapist carrying out the course of treatments, so the booking is best done by the therapist
An electrical treatment such as electrolysis	More thorough consultations and advice are needed before a client is allowed to have electrical treatments. Sometimes a doctor's permission is needed
A person under the age of 16 without a parent present	This is for insurance reasons, and to check that the client has parental permission
If a client cannot give you a contact telephone number	You would be unable to contact the client if there was a problem with the booking and you needed to change or cancel it, for example, due to staff illness
If a client comes in who has been disruptive and rude on a previous visit	A disruptive client will upset both staff and other clients

---

 REMEMBER

If at any time while helping on reception you are uncertain, you must ask for help. It isn't a sign of failure, it shows that you are acting sensibly.

 MEMORY JOGGER

1 How important is the reception?

2 How would you greet a client when she enters the reception?

3 Why is it important to read back the appointment details to the client after she has made a booking?

4 What problems could occur in the salon if the reception was badly run? ▼

MEMORY JOGGER

5 What details need to be written down when you take a message?

6 Give **four** reasons why a salon needs a reception area.

7 Give **four** positive and **four** negative methods of communication.

8 How would you deal with a client who starts to make a complaint in the reception area?

9 What are the booking codes and commercial timings for the following treatments?

   a a full leg wax

   b a manicure

   c a facial

   d a half leg wax and bikini line wax.

10 Explain the important points about the Data Protection Act.

11 What is meant by 'shelf life'?

12 How should make-up and skincare products be stored, so they are not ruined?

Section 3
TREATMENT ESSENTIALS

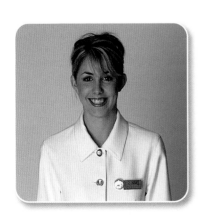
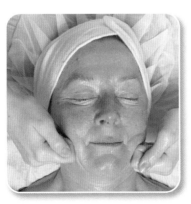
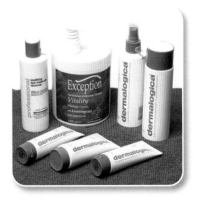

You, the beauty therapy assistant

Personal appearance

In Section 2, you studied the need for a beauty salon receptionist to have a professional appearance. This fact is also true when you are working as a beauty therapy assistant.

 CHECK IT OUT

Look back at the following sections:

① communication (pages 48–50)

② appearance and conduct (pages 44–46)

③ checklist for success (pages 44–45).

Consultation

 REMEMBER

A consultation is a question and answer session between you and your client. It enables you to find out information about your client. The consultation must be carried out before starting the treatment.

■ **Be neat!**

Write the information clearly on the record card, so that other members of staff can read your writing.

■ **Be polite!**

Show a friendly interest in your clients. Treat them with respect. Don't talk too loudly as all information the client gives you is confidential – the client may become embarrassed if she thinks that people can hear what is being said.

■ **Be aware!**

During the consultation you may discover that the client has **conditions** that you will need to work around, or more serious problems, called **contra-indications**, that you must not treat.

Contra-indications

A contra-indication is a condition that makes the client unsuitable for a treatment. If you carried out a treatment on a client with a contra-indication, it could spread an infection, make an illness worse, cause pain or result in a bad reaction.

■ If the contra-indication is nothing more serious than a bruise or a sore spot, the condition can be worked around.

■ However, if the contra-indication is more serious, for example, an infection, illness or *allergy*, **it must not be treated** until it has cleared up **or** a letter has been received from the client's doctor explaining that it is safe to treat.

A physical sensitivity to something that is eaten, a product used or something in the environment.

INFORMATION

A contra-indication that can be worked around and the treatment can be adapted for is **Local**.

A contra-indication that stops a treatment from being carried out is **Total**.

At Level 1, you will not be responsible for deciding if a client has a contra-indication and whether she can be treated. However, you must tell a senior therapist if you notice anything unusual.

 REMEMBER

The golden rule with consultations: when in doubt, check it out!

Health and hygiene

Remember to allow a small amount of time in between treatments to tidy and clean the treatment area, so that it is ready for the next client. It is bad practice for a client to enter a room or cubicle that is either unprepared, or is a mess of dirty towels and has products from the last treatment spread all over the trolley.

 REMEMBER

Tidy up as you go, it will save time later.

■ Replace bottle tops instantly.

■ Place waste in the bin straight away. This is also good practice with regard to Health and Safety, for example:
  ▪ nail varnish gives off very strong fumes
  ▪ used cotton wool and tissues contain germs.

■ During manicures and pedicures, use the nail varnish drying time to clear things away, for example, dirty towels and water in the manicure bowl. Clean tools and place them back in the steriliser.

■ During facials, use the time when the mask is on to tidy away small items and get fresh warm water – however, you must do this very quietly so as not to disturb the client.

Organising your workspace

Before starting a treatment, organise your work area so that everything is within reach and the trolley is set up with the necessary tools, equipment and products, as well as enough cotton wool and tissues. Your supervisor will show and advise you how to do this until you are able to set up on your own.

REMEMBER

It is bad practice to stop a treatment in order to fetch things. This breaks the flow of the treatment and is not relaxing for the client.

Setting up the workspace: a checklist

1. The client's record card and a pen should be on the trolley ready for the consultation.
2. The gown the client will wear during the treatment should be ready, and there should be a coat hanger or hook available for the client's clothes.
3. Clean towels should be laid out nearby, either on a stool or at the end of the couch.
4. The treatment couch should be prepared with a fitted bottom sheet and a disposable couch roll.
5. The trolley tops and work surfaces should be sanitised and covered with fresh couch roll.
6. The lotions and potions to be used during the treatment should be laid out on the trolley top.
7. The tools to be used during the treatment should be sterilised and then placed on the trolley top in a jar filled with antiseptic.
8. There should be enough cotton wool and tissues on the trolley to complete the whole treatment.

INFORMATION

It helps to have a checklist of all the tools, lotions and potions, and face/nail basics on a record card that you can keep nearby, for reference. Cover the list with a plastic cover so that it doesn't get marked, or have it laminated so that you can wipe it clean.

 REMEMBER

When you have finished the treatment, make sure that you leave the workspace perfect. It may help if you take a mental photograph of the area before you set up, for example, remember where and how everything was before you started and then put it back exactly how it was.

Preparing a client for treatment
Introductions

When the client is brought through to you, or you go to collect her from reception, make sure that you have an open, confident expression. Smile and make eye contact. Greet the client by her name, then introduce yourself and explain that you will be carrying out her treatment. Ask the client to follow you through to the treatment room. Before the treatment begins, make polite conversation to build a good relationship and help the client to feel at ease.

- Polite conversation is:
  - have you visited us before?
  - do you have regular treatments?
  - enquiring about other treatments the client has had in the past
  - is this treatment for a special occasion?
  - asking questions about the client's holidays or family
  - discussing the weather or light news topics.
- Polite conversation is **not**:
  - ignoring the client in order to talk to other members of staff
  - talking about yourself or another person, and not asking the client about herself
  - moaning about your last client or your job
  - telling the client your life story and about your problems at home
  - discussing serious news topics, religion or politics.

Client care

Remove and hang up the client's coat, then show her to her seat. Make sure that she is comfortable and provide help where necessary.

Client protection

Protect the client's clothes with a towel or gown. Be especially careful that she is protected from varnish or other products that might stain her clothes. For protection, roll up the client's sleeves to the elbow and then tuck tissue around them.

Just before you start

Ask the client to remove her jewellery and show her the bowl in which you will be placing it. Point out that, if she prefers, the client (not you) could put the jewellery in her handbag.

Sanitisation

Explain to the client that you are going to wash your hands as this gives her confidence in your cleanliness. Make sure that you dry your hands thoroughly, because wet hands are not clean hands.

Massage

The blood flow around the body.

Massage is relaxing and makes the client feel good. It is also good for the *circulation*, and therefore helps to improve skin colour and texture, and strengthens the nails.

INFORMATION

For Level 1, it is not necessary that you follow a set massage routine using all the movements. However, it is important that you carry out some sort of massage pattern that is relaxing for the client.

Massage has *three* main movements:

▪ **Effleurage**

This is a gentle stroking movement. It is used at the beginning or end of a treatment, or to join up other movements. It has a soothing and relaxing effect.

▪ **Petrissage**

These movements are circular or kneading movements. The hands, thumbs or fingertips are used to apply pressure to the muscles by lifting, rolling and pushing.

▪ **Tapotement**

This is a more stimulating movement in which the fingers, sides or palms of the hands produce light tapping, quick pinching or gentle slapping movements.

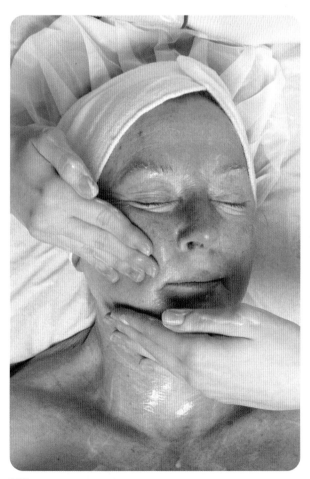

Effleurage movements

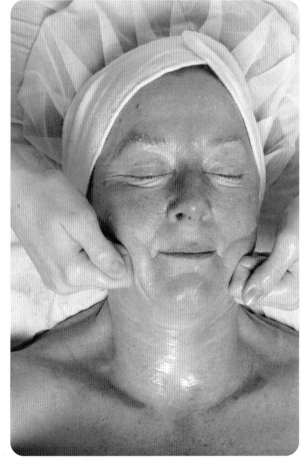

Petrissage movements

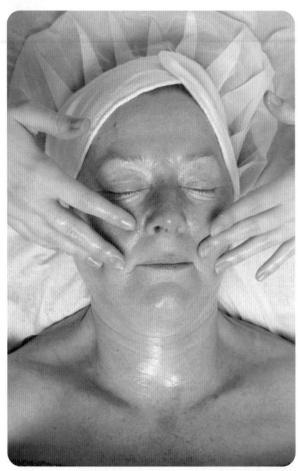

Tapotement movements

Treatment times and prices

The length of time it takes to carry out a facial or manicure can vary depending on the experience of the therapist and the condition of the client's skin and nails. However, the recommended times for basic treatments that are commercially acceptable are shown below. Prices can also vary a great deal. A central London salon is likely to be more expensive than one in a small market town and prices will vary according to where the treatment is taking place, e.g. a high street salon, day spa or top-class hotel.

▪ A Level 1 facial should take about 45 minutes. The cost of a salon facial to include massage of the face, neck and shoulders can vary from £20–40

▪ A Level 1 manicure should take about 30 minutes. The cost of a salon manicure to include massage of the hands and arms up to the elbow can vary from £12–25.

 CHECK IT OUT

Visit some salons, spas and health clubs – gather some of their price lists and display in your portfolio a price list for a salon at the lower end of the price scale and a price list for a salon at the higher end of the price scale. Which salons do you think offer value for money. Remember that the highest price is not always the best!

Section 4
PRACTICAL SKILLS

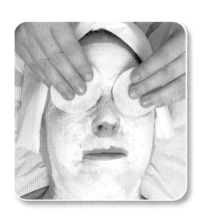
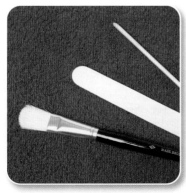
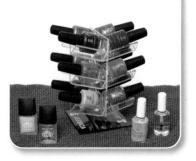

Introduction

In this unit, you will learn how to help with facial treatments. You will also learn about ways to improve the skin through the correct use of skincare products. In order to do this skilfully and confidently, you will need to show that you can:

- prepare your work area and client for treatment
- carry out a *consultation*
- carry out a facial treatment
- give advice on skincare.

A question and answer session to find out information about your client.

Saving face

Facial skin goes through many changes over the years. Our faces are under constant pressure from the weather and dirt in the environment, and also undergo a natural ageing process. Only some of us are lucky enough to have a naturally clear *complexion* that will not become too lined as we get older. We can cover up other parts of our body if they are less than perfect, however, this is not so with our faces. Our faces are on show all the time and it is therefore important that we look after them.

Good skin tone, texture and colour.

 REMEMBER

When you are young, it is easy to take the skin you have for granted. However, the steps you take now to look after your face will result in better skin when you are older. Don't leave your skincare until your face really needs it. Start now by carrying out gentle and careful cleansing, toning and moisturising.

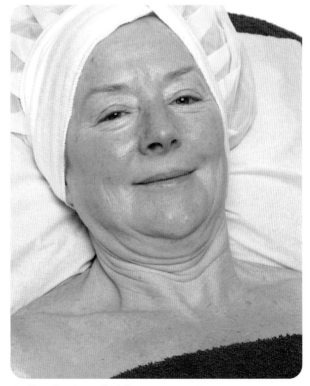

A client having a facial

Reasons why a client might want a facial:

Thirsty, lacking in water.

- For relaxation and a feeling of wellbeing.
- To add moisture to dry or *dehydrated* skin.

Marks on skin or bad skin conditions.

- To help clear spots and *blemishes*.
- To reduce the oil on greasy skin.

In this unit, you will cover the following topics:

- face file
- preparing to treat
- carry out a facial
- face follow-up.

Face file

What you will learn about:
- What is a facial?
- Layers of the skin
- Functions of the skin
- Muscles and bones of the face
- Skin health
- Skin types
- Spots
- Skin facts

What is a facial?

A facial is a treatment for the face and neck that lasts about one hour. It includes several smaller treatments that are carried out to:

Tiny openings in the skin that produce oil to moisturise the skin.

- deep clean the *pores*
- nourish and re-hydrate the skin
- relax the muscles
- improve the circulation
- brighten the complexion.

A facial includes:

Activity	Reason
A skin inspection	To find out skin type and problem areas
Cleansing and toning	To clean the skin
Exfoliation	To get rid of the dry, dead skin cells and freshen the complexion
Steaming	To relax the pores so they are easier to clean out
Comedone extraction	To remove blackheads with a special tool called a comedone extractor
Massage	To ease aching muscles, improve the blood flow and relax the client
Mask	To deep clean the skin and pores further
Moisturise	To soften and protect the skin

After a facial, the client should feel relaxed and her skin should glow.

Layers of the skin

The upper layer of the skin (epidermis) is made up of five layers. Each layer has a different job to do in order to keep the skin healthy. It is not essential that you know about the five layers of skin at Level 1, however, it may be useful to understand a little about them.

Look at the table below. You may find it easier to remember and say the English names rather than the Latin ones. It may also be helpful to know that 'stratum' is the Latin word for 'layer'.

The five layers of the epidermis are:

	Latin name	English name
Layer 1	Stratum Corneum	Horny layer
Layer 2	Stratum Lucidum	Clear layer
Layer 3	Stratum Granulosum	Granular layer
Layer 4	Stratum Spinosum	Prickle cell layer
Layer 5	Stratum Germinativum	Basal cell layer

Functions of the skin

Protection

Skin is like a waterproof jacket – it provides the body with protection from dirt, bacteria and injury. To keep the outer layers of skin smooth and soft, and free of splits and cracks that would let germs enter, the body produces oil through the skin's pores.

Sense and feeling

The nerve endings in our skin are very sensitive. They pick up changes in temperature or pressure, and alert us to pain. Messages are quickly sent from the nerve endings to our brain, so that we can respond – for example, by stopping the source of the pain.

The five layers of the epidermis

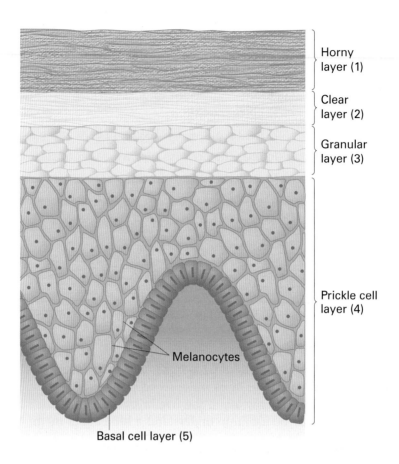

Horny layer (1)

Clear layer (2)

Granular layer (3)

Prickle cell layer (4)

Melanocytes

Basal cell layer (5)

Heat control

Skin helps to control the temperature in our body – how hot or cold we are.

- When we are too hot, we begin to sweat through sweat glands in our skin, and this cools us down.

- When we are too cold, the muscles that are joined to the hairs in our skin causes goose pimples and we begin to shiver, which warms up the body.

The correct temperature of the skin should be about 36°C.

Vitamin making

When we are outside, the sun's rays on the skin produce Vitamin D for the body. This vitamin is needed for strong bones and teeth.

Storage

The skin stores fat and water, without which we could not survive.

Waste removal

Poisons.

Some waste products and **toxins** are removed from the body through our sweat.

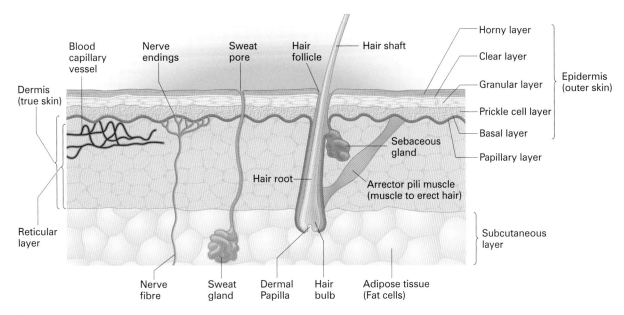

The structure of the skin

Muscles and bones of the face

Underneath the skin are muscles and bones.

- Each muscle adds shape to the face. Muscles also allow for facial movement, and each facial muscle produces a different movement.
- The bones provide support for the muscles and protect the brain and facial organs from injury.

Muscles of the face and neck

For Level 1, you do not need to know the correct names and actions of the muscles. However, the diagrams on page 88 will help you to understand the face better when you carry out practical treatments.

Bones of the face and skull

The bones of the face and skull keep the muscles of the head in place and protect the brain and other parts of the head from injury. There are twelve bones in the head in total.

The skull is made up of five bones.

> ### CHECK IT OUT
>
> **Funny faces**
> In pairs, look at the twelve different facial expressions on page 88. See if you can work out which muscles are being used for each expression. It will help if you make faces at each other.

Bone	Position
1 Occipital (x1)	At the back of the skull
2 Parietal (x2)	Positioned at the back of the head, and forms the roof of the skull
3 Frontal (x1)	Forms the front of the skull, forehead and upper eye sockets
4 Temporal (x1)	At the side, around the ears

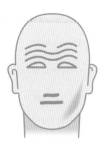

1. FRONTALIS
Amazement,
wonder,
shock

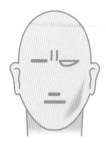

2. ORBICULARIS OCULI
Deep thought

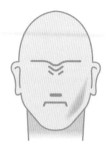

3. PROCERUS
Threatening,
unfriendliness,
anger

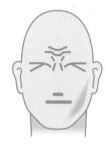

4. CORRUGATOR
Sadness and sorrow,
regret

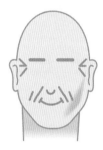

5. ZYGOMATICUS MAJOR
Laughter

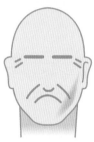

6. LEVATOR LABII SUPERIORIS
Grief, discontented

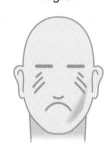

7. LEVATOR LABII
Extreme grief with
tears

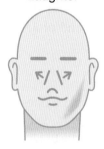

8. COMPRESSOR NARIS
Concentration, interest and
attention or anger and violent behaviour

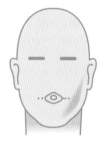

9. ORBICULARIS ORIS
Pouting, smoking,
kissing

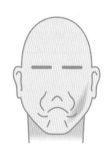

10. DEPRESSOR ANGULIORIS
Dislike, disapproval

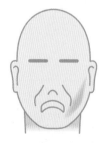

11. DEPRESSOR LABII INFERIORIS
Disgust

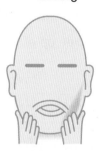

12. PLATYSMA
Anger, pain, torture
or hard work

The actions of different facial muscles in facial expression

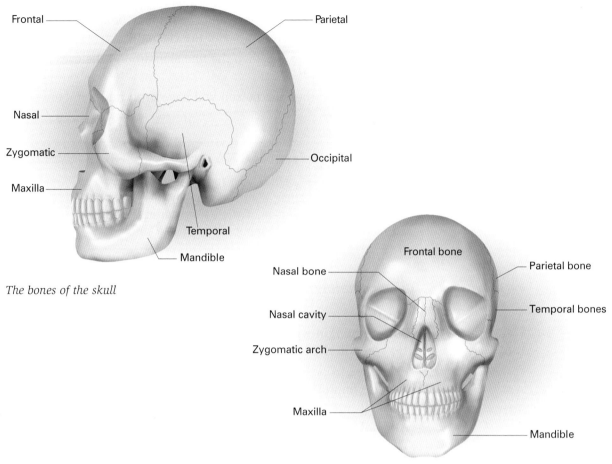

The bones of the skull

The bones of the face

The face is made up of seven bones.

Bone	Position
1 Zygomatic (x2)	These form the cheek bones
2 Maxilla (x2)	These form the upper jaw, most of the side wall of the nose and the front part of the soft palate (the top inside of the mouth)
3 Mandible (x1)	This is the lower jaw and is the only moving bone in the face. It enables movement of the mouth, for chewing and taking
4 Nasal (x2)	These form the bridge (upper part) of the nose

Skin health

Like the nails, the skin on the face reveals how healthy we are. It also shows how we feel – when we are fed up, stressed or have an illness, the skin becomes dull and lifeless. As we get older, facial skin can reveal the sort of life we have lived, for example, if a person has:

▪ **sunbathed** too much, the skin will be thickened, orangey yellow and very lined

- **smoked**, the skin around the mouth will have lines from sucking on the cigarette, and the nose and cheeks may be red with broken veins from the heat and smoke of the cigarette
- **cried or laughed a lot**, then the fine skin around the eyes can be very wrinkled
- **frowned a lot**, then the person will have deep ridges in between their eyebrows.

 CHECK IT OUT

Look closely at members of your family, for example, your baby sister, mother, aunt and grandmother. What do you notice about their skin? Write down your observations and then discuss them in groups or with your tutor.

Tips for healthy skin

Sun protection factor.

- **Weather**
  Protect the skin with creams that contain a UV-filter (at least **SPF** 15) when in the sun, and use a rich moisturiser in cold weather.
- **Exercise**
  Exercise improves the body's circulation – the blood flow around the body – which in turn improves the skin's colour and texture.

Vitamins and minerals.

- **Alcohol and drugs**
  These cause dehydration, which dries out the skin. They also result in the body losing important **nutrients** that the skin needs to work properly.
- **Smoking**
  Smoking ages and dries out the skin, and causes tiny broken blood vessels to appear. If you don't smoke, stay away from smoky areas.
- **Cleansing**
  It is important to keep the skin clean by cleansing every day. This prevents germs from building up and causing an infection. In addition, a dirty complexion is unattractive and looks unhealthy.
- **Sleep**
  It is important that you get plenty of sleep, because when you sleep your skin rests and repairs itself.
- **What you eat**
  It is important to eat a balanced diet that includes lots of fresh fruit and vegetables, and all of the vitamins and minerals that your body needs.

Dirt and germs that can cause bad health and poor skin.

- **Water**
  Drink lots of water daily – about 8 glasses. Water flushes out **impurities** from the body, which helps to keep the skin clear and prevents it from drying out.

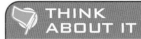

■ **For ageing**

As the skin gets older it loses moisture and *elasticity*, so it is important to take care of the skin from a young age by using moisturisers and gentle skin care.

Stretchiness.

Skin types

There are four main skin types:

■ normal

■ dry

■ oily

■ combination.

Each of the four skin types can also be:

■ sensitive – skin that easily becomes red, itchy and very dry

■ mature – older skin

■ dehydrated – skin lacking in water

■ congested – skin that has blocked pores and blemishes.

Deciding on a client's skin type is essential before you can decide on the best treatment for that client's skin. This is not always a simple process – it can take several years to master each part of a facial treatment and become an expert. However, for Level 1 only background knowledge of the basics is required. Let's take a closer look at skin types.

Normal skin

Normal skin is a rare skin type. It is usually found in children and young clients. It is smooth and clear with no blemishes. It feels soft to touch and has very tiny pores that are difficult to see. This type of skin needs lots of gentle care to keep it normal.

Dry skin

Dry skin is lacking in oil and may flake and chap easily. It can feel tight after washing, especially if soap is used. Dry skin absorbs creams and lotions easily, and can become lined and wrinkled early (especially around the eyes) unless it is *moisturised* well. Poor diet or not drinking enough water can cause dry skin or make it worse.

Softened and re-hydrated by the use of creams.

Oily skin

Oily skin is caused when too much oil is produced in the skin. Although we need oil to keep the skin smooth, when the body produces too much oil, this causes problems. Oily skin has a shiny complexion with lots of blackheads and blemishes. The pores are quite large and the skin can be quite thick. An oily skin can start or become worse as a teenager, when *puberty hormones* are most active.

Chemicals in the body that cause sexual development.

> **THINK ABOUT IT**
>
> Think about your lifestyle and the way in which you look after your skin. Will it lead to a healthy skin in later life? What things do you do that have an effect – good or bad – on your skin?

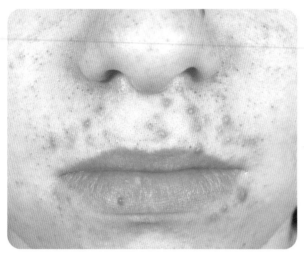

Blackheads

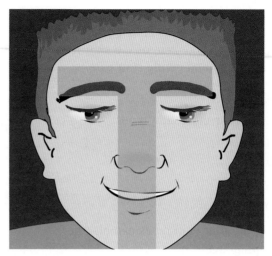

The T-zone

Combination skin

Combination skin is made up of two skin types. These types vary but the most common is a normal or dry skin on the cheek area, and an oily part on the nose and across the forehead (known as the T-zone). The oily T-zone shows up as a shiny nose and blackheads on the T-section.

> **✎ CHECK IT OUT**
>
> **What skin type are you?**
> Take a close look at your skin in the mirror. Use a good
> light and decide what skin type you have.
> Next, pair up with a friend and inspect each other's skin.
> Did you both agree on the skin type?

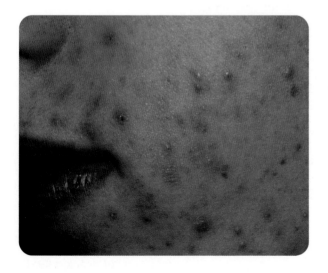

Spots

Spots, or acne, can be upsetting and are the curse of many people. They tend to form on oily skins. In most cases, spots can be prevented by good hygiene. However, if they do not clear up, there are alternative ways of treating them.

Acne vulgaris

The dos and don'ts of dealing with spots

Do:

- wash and dry your hands thoroughly before touching your skin
- clean your face thoroughly and remove all make-up before going to bed
- use a moisturiser to protect it from weather, dirt and dust
- treat your face gently – harsh products just make a problem worse, especially with sensitive or oily skin
- wear a sun protection cream, at least SPF 15
- exfoliate the skin regularly to remove dry or flaky skin on the surface that can block the pores

---

INFORMATION

The importance of exfoliating

Exfoliation gets rid of the dead dry skin on the surface which can block the outside of the hair follicles. These follicles become sticky when they become partly blocked with dead skin and **sebum**, resulting in blackheads and possibly more serious spots if left untreated.

Oil that is produced to keep the skin soft and supple.

Don't:

- go to bed with your make-up on
- pick dried spots – soften them with a moisturiser and leave them to heal naturally
- squeeze spots with dirty hands and fingernails
- sunbathe without a high factor sun cream – avoid sunburn and sunbeds
- use strong spot creams and lotions – these are very stimulating to the oil glands, so your skin will produce more oil instead of less

Skin facts

1. The upper layer of the epidermis is dead skin cells.
2. Skin is constantly flaking off. This is to allow for new skin underneath to replace it.
3. The inner layers of skin are constantly moving up and replacing the outer layers of skin that have been shed.
4. Skin takes about 28 days to renew itself completely.
5. Skin becomes drier as we get older.
6. The condition of the skin varies with the time of year and the weather, and your health and age.
7. The skin is the largest organ of the body – it provides an unbroken covering over the body.

8 The skin is very elastic and can stretch to fit the size of your body.

9 Skin is thinnest on the eyelids (less than 0.5 mm) and thickest (6 mm or more) on the soles of the feet.

10 The skin protects our body and is sensitive to heat, cold and pain.

INFORMATION

Protecting the skin from the sun
Skin cancer is on the increase, so sunbathe and use sunbeds in moderation. If out in the sun, always use the correct factor sun cream for your skin type.

At a gently sloping angle.

Prepare to treat!

What you will learn about:

■ Prepare yourself

■ The workspace

■ Client consultation

■ Lotions and potions

■ Face basics

■ Tech tools

Prepare yourself

CHECK IT OUT

Review Section 3: Treatment Essentials (pages 75–80).

The workspace
Where and how?

A facial treatment is typically carried out while a client lies on a comfortable couch. The client may lie completely flat or *semi-inclined*.

Posture and lighting

Posture
You will need to decide whether you will stand or sit behind the couch. It depends on:

■ the height and angle of the couch – whether it's flat or sloping

■ your height and whether you can reach the client if you sit down.

It is very important that you do not overstretch your neck and back to reach the client's face because you will end up with a long-term back problem. Overstretching will also affect the muscles and veins in your legs and could possibly cause varicose veins over time.

> **REMEMBER**
>
> When standing for long periods, move a little to keep the circulation going. For example, every now and then:
> - move from one foot to the other
> - bend the knee back a few times, then repeat on the other foot.

Bad posture will cause physical aches and pains. In addition, the treatment will probably not be as good because it has been carried out in an awkward position. The client will also suffer, as the treatment that was meant to be relaxing and enjoyable can end up being uncomfortable.

Lighting

Lighting must be bright and clear for the skin inspection, but soft and relaxing for the rest of the facial treatment. A light that can be dimmed is ideal, along with a magnifying lamp for the inspection.

Health and hygiene

The differences between sanitisation, disinfection and sterilisation were covered in Section 2 (pages 28–29). Let's now think about the practical side of health and hygiene for facial treatments. The table below shows how **cross-infection** can occur during a facial treatment and why.

When germs or bacteria are transferred from one person to another.

Potential cross-infection during a facial treatment

Facial activity	What could happen	How infections could start
The therapist has not washed her hands before the treatment	Illness and skin infections	- The therapist goes to the toilet and then continues the treatment - The therapist has completed a treatment on one client and then carried straight on to the next client
Removing blackheads	Skin infections and spread of germs	The blackhead extractor has not been sterilised
Applying a mask	Skin and eye infections and spread of germs	The mask brush has not been washed and sterilised
Applying moisturiser	Skin infections and spread of germs	The therapist uses her fingers to scoop out the cream from the pot instead of a disposable spatula. After a few treatments, the cream is full of germs from different clients

REMEMBER

The results of cross-infection are horrible, so make sure that you always **follow the correct hygiene methods** when giving a treatment. The results of not being hygienic could be very damaging for both the salon and your career.

Client consultation

 CHECK IT OUT

Review Section 3: Treatment Essentials (pages 75–76).

At first, you will watch and learn from the therapist while she is carrying out a consultation. Eventually, you will have gained enough experience to carry out the consultation yourself under the supervision of the therapist.

 REMEMBER

A client consultation should be carried out using questioning, visual and manual methods. You will need to listen and respond very carefully.

The information that you need to find out from a client before carrying out a facial treatment is:

Name

It is best to have a record of both the client's first name and surname. It is important to record the first name because there could be two clients with the same surname. If you only write the surname, this could cause confusion and client records may become mixed up.

Address

Write the client's full address including postcode.

Telephone number

Always write down a home number and a work or mobile number. One telephone number is not enough – if a client's appointment needs to be cancelled at short notice, you will not be able to contact her if she is at work and you only have her home telephone number!

The client's reason for the facial and her needs/wishes for today

Asking this information of your client will help you to understand what she needs from her facial treatment, for example, whether it is a deep cleansing maintenance or a relaxing, de-stressing treatment.

Condition of skin when inspected

When you carry out a consultation, you will need to find out information from your client by:

■ **Questioning**
This is when you ask the client questions about her skin, home skincare routine, problem areas and treatment requirements.

■ **Visual inspection**
This is when you look at the client's skin colour, texture, pore size and blemishes.

■ **Manual inspection**
This is when you feel the smoothness, softness, firmness and hydration of the client's skin.

All of these activities – questioning, visual and manual – will help you to build a picture of what the client needs from a facial treatment.

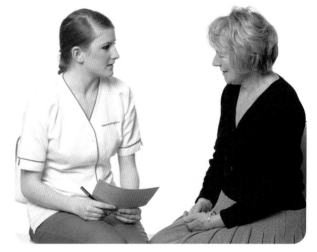

Questioning a client before a facial

Contra-indications and conditions

Are there any signs of skin or eye disorders or infections? If yes, then:

■ Can they be worked around if covered?

■ Are they a total contra-indication?

■ Will you be able to treat the client with her doctor's permission?

Products used during the facial

Which cleanser, toner and moisturiser did you use – for what skin type? Did you use eye cream or night cream? What ingredients were in the mask and what skin type was it? Write down as much information as possible about the products used during the facial.

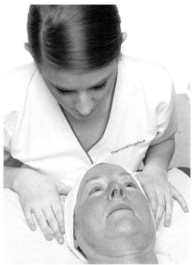

Performing a visual inspection before a facial

Homecare advice

What help and advice did you give your client on how she could improve the condition of her skin? When did you advise her to return for another salon treatment?

Product sales

Did you sell the client any skincare products or give her advice on what to buy for the future?

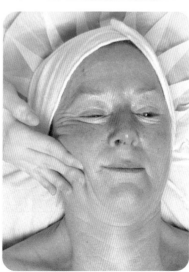

Carrying out a manual inspection before a facial

Comments

This is where you can write your thoughts about the treatment

▮ Were you happy with the result?

▮ Was the client pleased with her treatment?

▮ How did the client's skin look and feel after the treatment?

Record of treatments

Write the date, type of facial, the therapist's name, and any extra notes that may be useful in the future.

FACIAL CONSULTATION SHEET

DATE *10/4/03*   NAME *Miss N Shah*

ADDRESS *3 Oak Avenue, Newtown*

TELEPHONE NUMBER (H) *0208 976 1133* (W) *0207 612 1060*

CONDITION OF SKIN ON INSPECTION

Clear, complexion, fine lines around the eyes, a few broken capillaries on cheek area. Feels slightly dry.

CONTRA-INDICATIONS/CONDITIONS

No contra-indications. Comedones around nose and chin.

PRODUCTS USED

Nourishing Nature's range for dry skin.

HOMECARE ADVICE

Drink more water to re-hydrate the skin.

Use sunscreen and exfoliate weekly.

PRODUCT SALES

Nourishing Nature's trial pack for dry skin.

COMMENTS

Client was very relaxed and pleased with how her skin felt, has re-booked for a month's time.

RECORD OF TREATMENTS

DATE	TREATMENT	THERAPIST
10/4/03	*Facial*	*Lucy Brent*

A typical consultation card for a facial treatment

Contra-indications and conditions for facial treatments

 REMEMBER

At Level 1, you are not responsible for deciding if a client has a contra-indication or not. However, you must tell a senior therapist if you notice anything unusual.

You will need to look out for:

- splits or blisters around the nose and mouth that could be a cold sore
- bloodshot and watery eyes that could be an allergy or *conjunctivitis*
- dry, red and flaky skin, which could be *eczema or dermatitis*
- cuts or grazes that could cause cross-infection
- redness – it could be a sign of an allergy or an injury
- swelling or lumps – it could be bruising or something much more serious that needs to be checked by a doctor.

An eye infection.

Dry skin conditions that show up as rough, flaky skin. The skin becomes very sensitive and itchy and can be red and angry looking. In very bad cases, the skin leaks a watery fluid.

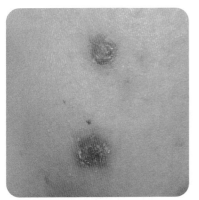

Skin infections – Impetigo

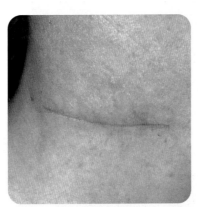

Cold sores

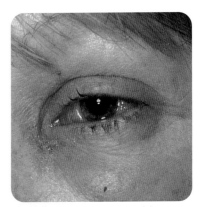

Eye infection – Conjunctivitis

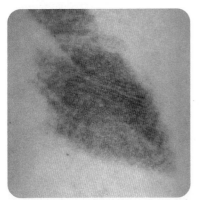

Bruising

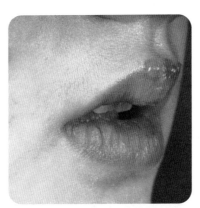

Scar tissue less than six months old

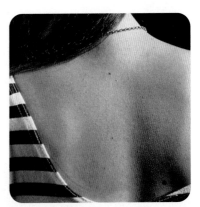

Recent sunburn

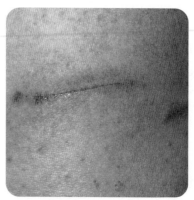

Cuts and grazes

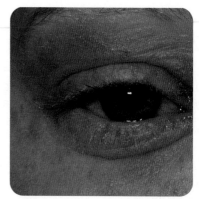

Eczema

Lotions and potions
Eye make-up remover

Purpose

To become a liquid.

These are mild cleaning products that ***dissolve*** eye make-up so that it can be easily wiped off without rubbing the eyes.

Types

Eye make-up remover is available as an oil, lotion or gel. Some remove waterproof make-up.

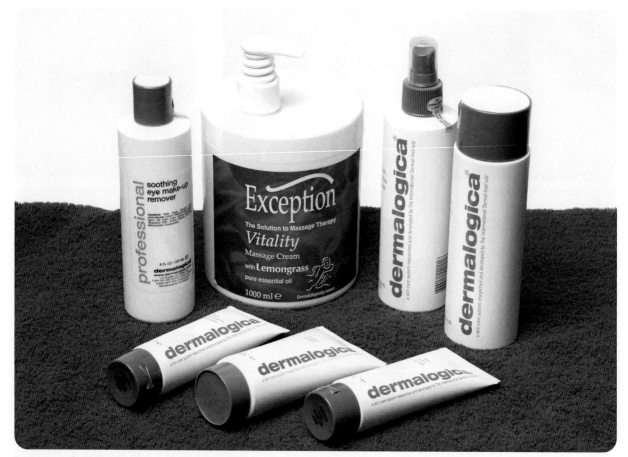

Lotions and potions used in a facial treatment

Cleansers

Purpose

- To remove old make-up.
- To clean dirt, dust and grime from the skin and pores.
- To remove oil and dead skin cells.

Types

- **Cream** – this thick, creamy cleanser is used for dry or mature skin types. It dissolves make-up quickly.
- **Milk** – this is a thin, runny cleanser that can be used on most skin types, except very dry skin. It is ideal for young or normal skin types, but is not very good at removing heavy or waterproof make-up.
- **Lotion** – this is similar in thickness to a milk cleanser but includes *anti-bacterial ingredients* to help spotty and combination skins, which are usually found in younger clients.
- **Facial washes** – these can be liquids, gels or lotions. They are gently rubbed into the skin with some water to make a *lather*. Facial washes can be used on any skin, as long as moisturiser is applied afterwards, as the skin can feel quite tight. Facial washes are especially good for men and people who like to feel freshly washed.

Ingredients to cut down the spread of germs and infections that could make a problem skin worse.

Foam and bubbles.

Toners

Purpose

- To remove any left-over cleanser from the skin.
- To dissolve oil.
- To refresh and cool the skin.
- To tighten the skin and pores.

Types

Toners come in different strengths and are chosen depending on the skin type. The main ingredients are water, alcohol, colour and perfume. The greater the alcohol content, the stronger the toner. Toners for oily problem skins are called **astringents** and have the highest alcohol content.

Face masks

For Level 1 you only need to know how to use a ready-made non-setting face mask, however, it is helpful if you have a basic knowledge of the other types that you might see being used in the salon.

Face masks are usually applied towards the end of a facial, after the skin has been cleansed, steamed and massaged. A mask should never be applied on skin that has not been thoroughly cleansed.

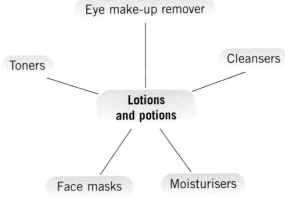

Different products for facial use

Purpose

Depending on the ingredients, face masks can:

- deep clean the skin and pores
- remove oil and dead skin cells
- deeply moisturise and nourish the skin
- tighten the pores
- soften fine lines
- soothe sensitive skins.

Types

- **Setting** – these masks are usually made of clay powder. They are mixed with distilled water or a toner to make a paste that can be painted on the skin with a mask brush.
- **Non-setting** – these masks can be creams or gels in a tube or pot.
- **Specialised** – these are nourishing warm oil masks or deeply moisturising paraffin wax masks.
- **Food** – Just as the name says, these face masks can be made using ingredients from your own fridge at home!

 CHECK IT OUT

Food masks
Why don't you try these recipes out?

- **For dry skin**
Mash avocado, add egg yolk and mix until creamy. Apply to the face with a spatula. Leave for 10–15 minutes, then clean off.

- **For oily skin**
Mix oatmeal and honey together, then apply to the face with a spatula. Leave for 10–15 minutes, then clean off.

When using food ingredients, you should use the masks as soon as you have made them, as they can go off very quickly.

Moisturiser

Purpose

- To soften and protect the skin's surface.
- To *re-hydrate* the skin.
- To help the application of make-up by providing a smooth base.

Adding water or moisture.

Types

As with cleansers, moisturisers can be:

- creams for dry skins
- lotions for oily skins
- milks for young, normal or sensitive skins.

What you will need

Before starting a treatment, essential preparation is needed to make sure that you are well prepared and have all the necessary equipment and products. In both the facial and nail units in Section 4, you will be provided with a list of what you will need under three headings. (Your tutor may at times wish to add a few items to the list, so check first.) These are:

- **Basics** – the disposable products, laundry and workspace requirements.
- **Tech tools** – the tools, such as tweezers and scissors, that you will need.
- **Lotions and potions** – all the products needed for the treatment (you have already covered these on pages 100–102).

Face basics

Dampened cotton wool

This is used for:

1. **Cotton wool squares** – for removing cleanser and putting on toner. They need to be large enough to wrap around your first two fingers.

2. **Cotton wool half moons** – these are placed under the bottom eyelashes, to protect the skin under the eyes from the make-up that is being cleansed off.

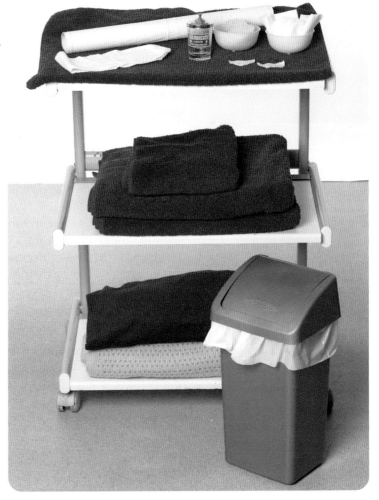

Face basics

③ **Eye pads (circles or squares)** – these rest on the eye while using the magnifying lamp for skin inspection or blackhead removal. They can be soaked in witch hazel to soothe the eyes while the client is wearing a face mask.

INFORMATION

How to prepare dampened cotton wool squares

❶ Cut squares approximately 3-inch in size from a cotton wool roll.

❷ Take about 4–6 squares and hold them between the palms of your hands under a running tap. When they are soaked through, squeeze out the water so that they are only damp and not dripping.

❸ Peel back thin layers from your thick pad of cotton wool. You should have about 16–20 pads. These are your facial pads for removing and applying products.

Dry cotton wool

This is used to cover the tip of an orange stick for removing eye make-up.

Tissues

Tissues are used for blotting excess toner or moisturiser. Tissues are normally 2-ply – this means that each tissue is made up of two very thin layers. For the purpose of beauty treatments, however, tissues are split as this makes them more economical to use and easier to curve around the shape of the face.

Sponges

These can be used with warm water to remove mask products from the skin. However, they are not easy to clean and sterilise. They need to be washed in very hot soapy water, dried thoroughly and then placed in an ultraviolet sterilising cabinet. The other option is for a salon to charge enough for a facial so that the sponge can be given to the client at the end of her treatment. Otherwise, it is best to use damp cotton wool squares for mask removal.

Towels

You will need one hand towel to dry your own hands during the treatment, one medium-sized towel for placing across the client's chest, and one large towel for covering her body during the treatment (if a blanket is not used).

Blanket

In the winter months, a honeycomb blanket may be needed to keep the client warm during the treatment.

INFORMATION

Each salon has its own way of preparing a client for a treatment, so you will need to find out how your workplace sets up – whether they use sheets and blankets, or towels.

Fitted couch sheet

This protects the couch from marks and product spills during a treatment.

Couch roll

This is used to cover the fitted couch sheet so that it doesn't need to be washed after each treatment. It is also used to protect the towel lying over the client's chest, the pillow and the headband from skincare and mask products.

Headband or turban

This is used to protect the client's hair from the products, and to prevent her hair from getting in the way of the treatment.

Gown

After the client has finished her consultation, you will need to ask her to remove her top clothing. If she has to go to a treatment **cubicle** to change, you will need to give her a gown to wear, to prevent any embarrassment. The gown is then removed when you help the client onto the couch to start her treatment.

Separate workspace or changing area.

Waste bin

A pedal bin with a lid is best for hygiene purposes, as you can open it without touching it with your hands.

Sterilising jar

This should be filled with antiseptic or disinfectant solution, so that small metal tools such as blackhead extractors and tweezers can be placed in it during the treatment. The solution will help to keep germ levels down, but it will not destroy germs completely. The solution should be changed after every client.

Dishes

Small plastic or metal dishes are needed to hold cotton wool and tissues, as well as the client's jewellery.

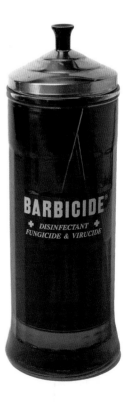

Sterilising jar

> **INFORMATION**
>
> If a client removes her jewellery and places it in the dish, the jewellery dish should then be placed on top of the trolley so that the client is able to see it at *all* times. This is for security reasons and it also acts as a memory jogger, so that the client doesn't forget her jewellery when she leaves.

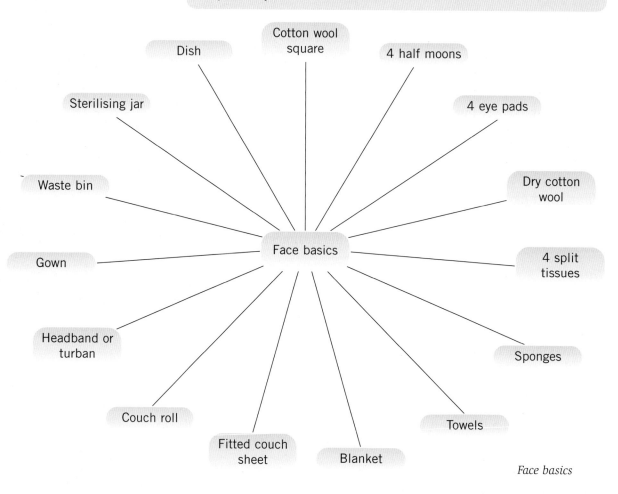

Face basics

Tech tools
Spatula

A spatula is a wide wooden stick that is used to scoop out cream or lotion from pots. Fingers should never be used, as this is very unhygienic and could result in cross-infection. A spatula is also used to tuck the client's hair into a headband instead of your fingers.

Orange sticks

These are made of orange wood, which is slightly bendy. One end is pointed and the other end is shaped like a hoof. Both ends of the orange stick are coated in cotton wool for hygiene purposes, as the cotton wool can be removed and thrown away after use. The cotton wool softens the tip for safety when cleaning around the eyes.

Comedone extractor

This loop-end tool is designed to remove blackheads. It is pressed onto a blackhead, then steady, gentle pressure is applied. If the blackhead is ready, its content will pop out.

Mask brush

This is usually a strong bristle brush that is used to paint the mask onto the skin. Some brushes are fan shaped. They are very hard to sterilise completely, so care must be taken to wash them thoroughly with hot soapy water, leave them to dry and then place them in an ultraviolet sterilising cabinet for the recommended time. Alternatively, a disposable spatula can be used to apply some masks.

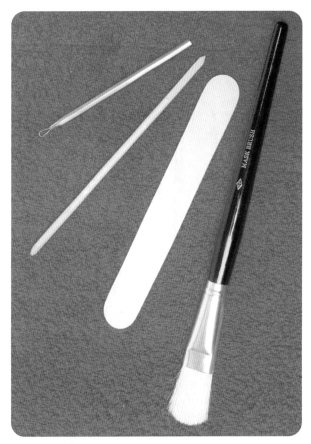

Tools for a facial treatment

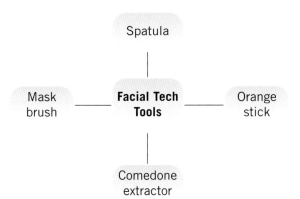

Tools used in facial treatments

 SALON STORY

During a consultation, Petra asked her client what she hoped to gain from today's facial. The client said that she had a big dinner party tonight and wanted to go out feeling like a 'new woman'. The client said that her skin was dry and flaky, and that her make-up wouldn't go on very smoothly. The client hoped that Petra would be able to improve the texture of her skin, so that her make-up looked great for tonight.

It was obvious to Petra that the client had not been advised as to what a facial is, and therefore had her heart set on:

■ a treatment for dry flaky skin
■ being able to apply great make-up for her dinner party.

❶ How could Petra explain the purpose of a facial to her client?

❷ What other choices could Petra give her client?

Write down or discuss how you would deal with these problems.

Carry out a facial

What you will learn about:

- Preparation and consultation
- Make-up removal
- Cleansing routine
- Tone and refresh
- Full skin inspection
- Exfoliation and massage
- The face mask
- Soften and smooth
- Face follow-up

You will see that each step of the facial is labelled numerically as you go through this section.

Preparation and consultation

Before you start:

- Make a quick check of your workplace preparation.
- Remove your watch, and your own and the client's jewellery.
- Wash your hands.
- Carry out the consultation.
- Assess the condition of your client's skin.
- Check for conditions and contra-indications.
- Ask the client to remove the clothes from her top half, take them and hang them up. Give the client a gown if necessary.
- Help the client on to the couch. Cover her with the blankets or towels, and ask her if she is warm and comfortable.

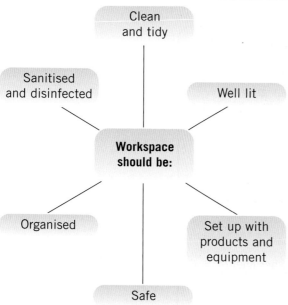

Workspace presentation

> **💡 REMEMBER**
>
> If you have carried out the consultation, ask a senior member of staff to double check that you have not overlooked any infection or problem.

> **INFORMATION**
>
> Throughout the facial, explain what you are doing and why because it is important to keep the client informed. Chat to the client about her wishes for today's treatment. Remember, the client's wishes can change from one week to the next, so check each time.

Preparing the client

1 Protect the client's hair with a headband. Tuck either tissue or couch roll under the headband to keep it as clean as possible. Place a medium-sized towel across the client's chest, then slip her bra straps down over her upper arms and tuck the towel over and under the straps, to protect them from the products.

Make-up removal

2 Place the half moons under the bottom lashes, ask client to close her eyes. Squeeze a small amount of cleanser on to a spatula. Using your index finger (first finger) dip it into the cleanser and gently rub on and around the eye in a circular movement.

3 Now use a covered orange stick to wipe away the make-up and cleanser. Use gentle downward strokes until the eye and lashes are free from make-up. Repeat on the other eye. Then ask the client to open her eyes so that you can clean underneath them.

4 Next, gently rub some cleanser onto the lips. Hold on one side of the mouth for support, then wipe the make-up away with the other hand using damp cotton wool. Then hold the other side of the mouth, and repeat.

> ### INFORMATION
>
> You may need to repeat the eye make-up removal process for very heavy or waterproof make-up.

Cleansing routine

The cleansing routine is carried out with gentle, upward massage movements. These are mainly **effleurage** (see page 79).

> **REMEMBER**
>
> For Level 1, it is not necessary for you to follow a set massage routine using all the movements. However, it is important to carry out some sort of pattern that is relaxing to the client. Below is a simple cleansing routine for you to follow.

5 Squeeze a small amount of cleanser into the palm of your hands – about the size of a 50-pence coin. Then put your hands together so that you have the cleanser in both hands. Gently press your hands over the face and neck of your client, to coat her skin in cleanser. Take care not to get any cleanser in her eyes and mouth.

6 Using gentle, upward effleurage strokes, distribute the cleanser evenly over the face.

STEP-BY-STEP FACIAL 1

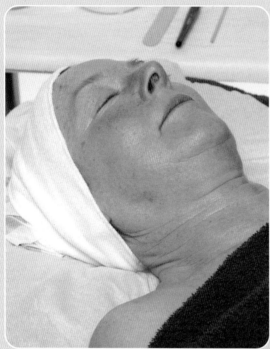

1 Prepare the client for her facial

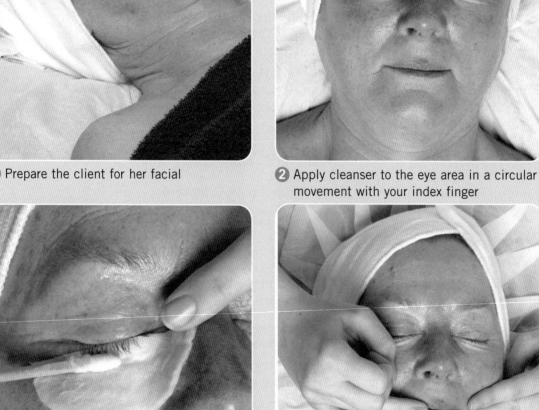

2 Apply cleanser to the eye area in a circular movement with your index finger

3 Use a covered orange stick to wipe away the make-up and cleanser. Use gentle downward strokes until the eye and lashes are free from make-up. Repeat on the other eye

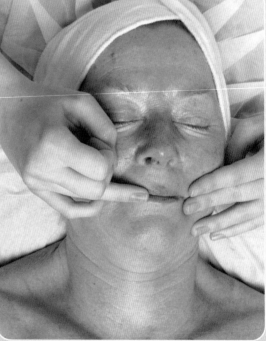

4 Gently rub some cleanser onto the lips to remove make-up

STEP-BY-STEP FACIAL 2

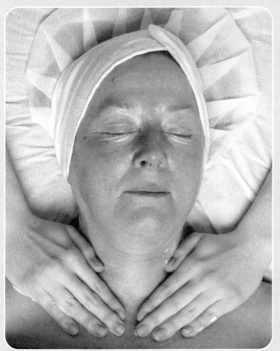

5 Squeeze a small amount of cleanser onto your hands. Gently press your hands over the client's face and neck to apply cleanser

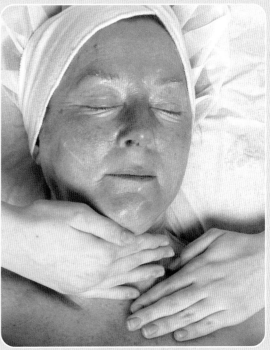

6 Use gentle, upward effleurage strokes to distribute the cleanser over the face

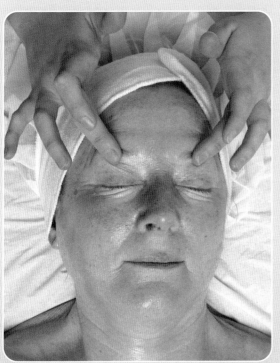

7 Spread the cleanser around the eyes using gentle circular movements.

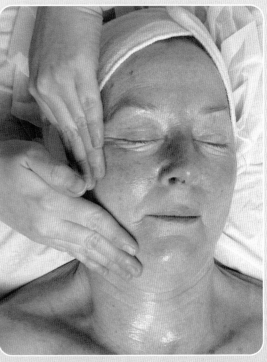

8 Use gentle upward effleurage strokes to spread the cleanser over the cheeks

7 Following the direction of the brows, gently circle the eyes with the middle fingers to distribute the cleanser.

8 Use gentle upward effleurage strokes to distribute the cleanser.

9 Now follow the cleansing routine shown in stages A to L, which is designed to thoroughly cleanse the client's neck and face. *All* movements are done lightly and your hands *must never* leave the client's skin.

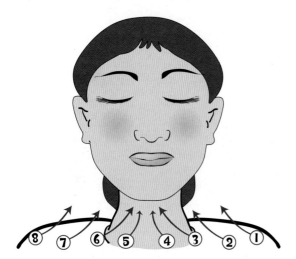

A: Eight upward strokes of the shoulders, chest area and neck with the palms of the hands. Start with the left side and gradually work to the right side

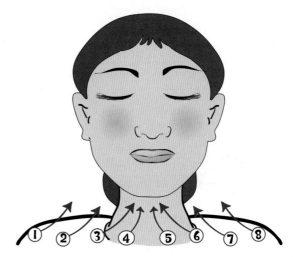

B: Repeat stage A, this time working from the right to the left side

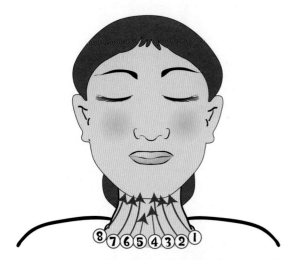

C: Eight upward strokes of the neck with the palms of the hands. Start with the left side and gradually work to the right side

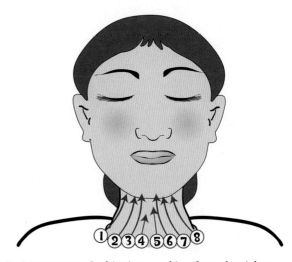

D: Repeat stage C, this time working from the right to the left side

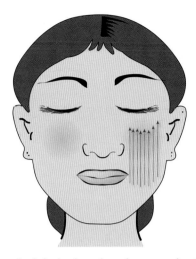

E: Slide to the left cheek and stroke upwards eight times

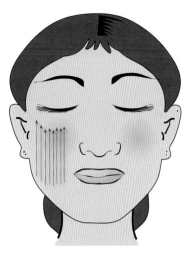

F: Then slide to the right cheek and stroke upwards eight times

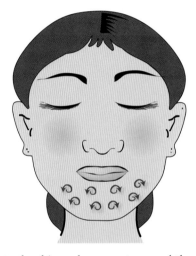

G: Slide to the chin and carry out upward thumb circles eight times

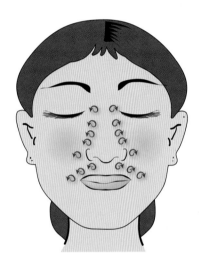

H: Using middle and index fingers, circle eight times under and around the sides of the nose

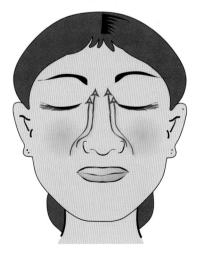

I: Slide up to the bridge of the nose and stroke upwards four times

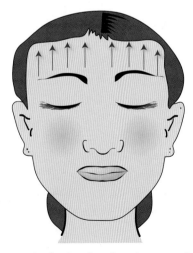

J: Slide up to the forehead and stroke upwards eight times, moving from the left to the right and then back again

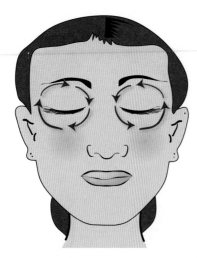

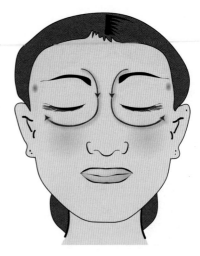

K: Slide your hands to the middle of the forehead and circle the eyes gently four times in the direction of growth of the eyebrow

L: Slide to the temples and apply gentle pressure, to complete the routine

10 Take two damp cotton wool squares and wrap them around your first two fingers.

11 Remove the cleanser, which has now mixed with the dirt and face make-up. Use exactly the same strokes as for the cleansing diagrams (step 9).

12 Carry out a second cleanse by repeating steps 5–10.

Tone and refresh

13 Take two more damp cotton wool squares and soak them in toning lotion. Repeat steps 10 and 11 with toner instead of cleanser, to tone the skin and remove the last traces of cleanser.

14 Take a split tissue and place it on the client's face, to blot the toning lotion. Fold it down from the forehead to the lower face and then onto the neck. Take two more split tissues and blot the chest and each shoulder.

15 Tone the skin a second time by repeating steps 13 and 14.

Full skin inspection

16 Your client's skin should be completely clean, dry and grease free. Now carry out a thorough skin inspection under the magnifying lamp.

Assessing the condition

When carrying out the skin inspection, make notes on the record card under the following headings:

Skin disorders and contra-indications
Look out for signs of these, which were covered on page 99.

Skin colour

- Does it have a healthy glow?
- Are there areas of redness that could suggest sensitivity?
- Is the skin tanned or is it a yellowy colour?

STEP-BY-STEP FACIAL 3

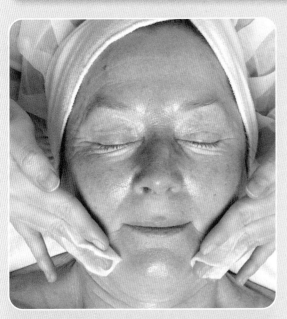

9 & 10 Once you have followed the cleansing routine (stages A–L) on pages 112–14, wrap two cotton wool squares around your first two fingers.

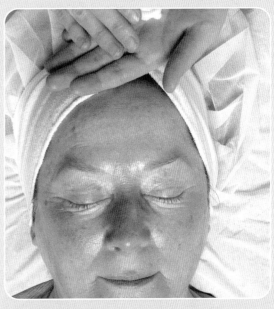

11&12 Remove cleanser with damp cotton wool using exactly the same strokes as for cleansing (step 9). Carry out a second cleanse by repeating steps 5–10.

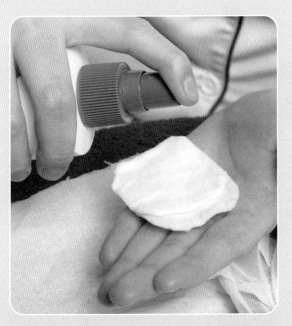

13 Take two more damp cotton wool squares and soak them in toning lotion. Repeat steps 10 and 11 with toner instead of cleanser, to tone the skin and remove the last traces of cleanser

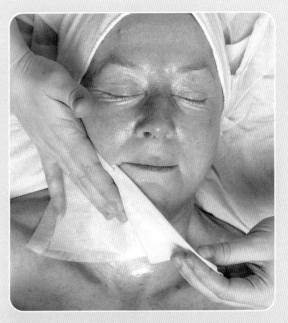

14 &15 Using a split tissue, blot the toning lotion. Tone the skin a second time by repeating steps 13 and 14

STEP-BY-STEP FACIAL 4

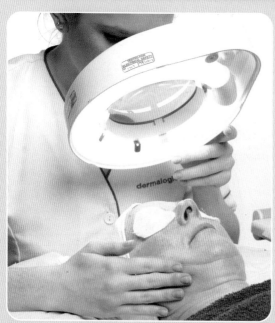

16 Carry out a skin inspection under the magnifying lamp

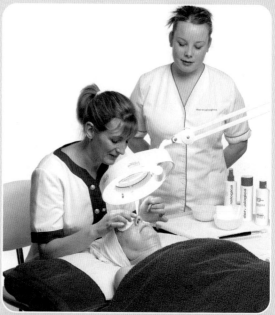

17 The senior therapist will carry out a skin exfoliating treatment, steam and comedone extraction. After extraction, tone and blot the skin

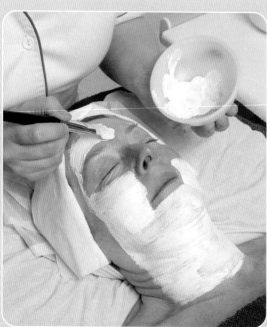

18 After the senior therapist has completed the massage, apply the face mask evenly taking care to avoid the lips, eyes, nostrils and hairline

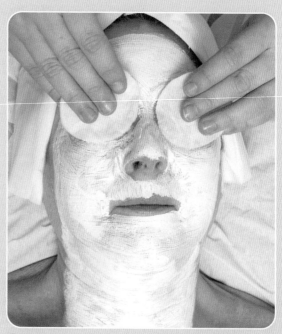

19 After the face mask has been applied, place eye circles over your client's eyes, then leave her to rest and relax for about 10 minutes

Skin texture

Touch the skin. How does it feel?

- Soft or rough?
- Dry or oily?
- Flaky or smooth?
- Thin or thick?
- Firm or loose?

Skin and muscle tone

- Is the skin young and firm with good muscle tone and tight skin?
- Is the skin around the eyes and mouth loose with lines and wrinkles?
- Are there frown lines on the forehead?

The eyes

- Are there laughter lines around the eyes? These are called '**crow's feet**'.
- Are there dark circles or puffiness around or under the eyes?

The T-zone

Is the T-zone shiny with blackheads, spots and open pores?

Client information

- Ask the client:
  - what products does she use on her skin?
  - what is her normal skincare routine?

Exfoliation and massage

⑰ Next, the senior therapist will carry out a skin exfoliating treatment, steam and comedone extraction. After extraction, tone and blot the skin by repeating steps 13 and 14.

The senior therapist will now massage the client's face, neck and shoulders. The massage should last about 15–20 minutes.

Massage is a very skilful part of the facial treatment and can take a long time to master, so make sure that you watch the senior therapist carefully. As you become more skilled at your treatment, you may be allowed to carry out part of the massage.

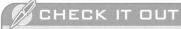 **CHECK IT OUT**

While you are learning about massage, try practising some movements on another therapist so that she can give you feedback on how to improve.

The face mask

Before applying the face mask, make sure that your client's skin is free of oils and creams. Then choose a pre-prepared, non-setting mask to suit your client's skin type.

18 Place enough of the mask in a bowl to coat the whole of your client's face and neck. Then, using a mask brush, paint the mask onto the skin. Start at the neck and move upwards in smooth strokes. Continue up the face applying a good even covering, and finish with the forehead. Do not apply the mask to the lips, eyes, nostrils and hairline, and take care to avoid these areas.

19 When you have finished applying the face mask, place dampened eye circles over your client's eyes. Allow the client to rest and relax for about 10 minutes, depending on the manufacturer's instructions for the face mask.

 REMEMBER

Always follow the manufacturer's instructions when using beauty products. The instructions should have information about
- how to use the product
- how long to leave it on the skin
- how to store it
- how to use it safely.

20 After your client has rested with the face mask on for about 10 minutes, remove the eye pads. Then press damp sponges all over the mask, allowing the water from the sponges to soak into the mask.

21 Now remove the face mask with firm upward strokes. Start at the neck, and work up over the cheeks and onto the nose and forehead. Continue until all the mask is removed. Use fresh warm water, if necessary.

 REMEMBER

It is very important to check that every trace of the mask is removed – make sure that no mask remains anywhere on the skin. Check behind the ears and under the chin.

22 Finally, repeat steps 13 and 14 to tone and blot the skin. Make sure the skin is dry.

STEP-BY-STEP FACIAL 5

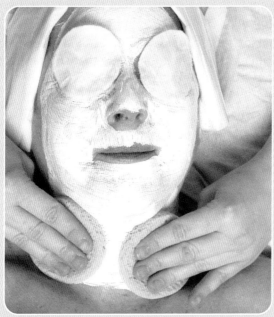

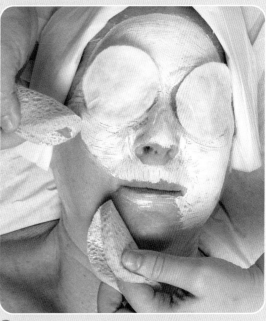

20 After 10 minutes remove the eye pads and press damp sponges over the mask, allowing the water to soak in

21 Starting at the neck and working up over the cheeks onto the nose and forehead, remove all the face mask with firm upward strokes

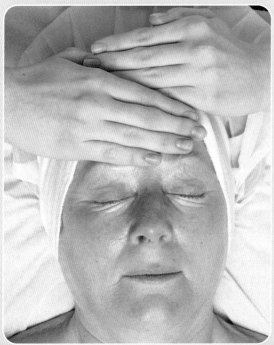

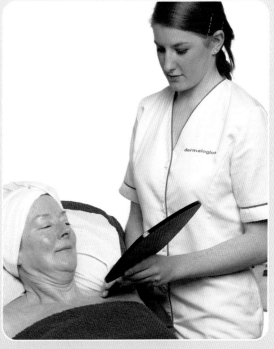

22&23 Tone and blot the skin. Apply moisturiser for the correct skin type using the cleansing routine on pages 112–14. Blot the skin if there is too much moisturiser on it

24 Offer the client a mirror so that she can check her complexion

Soften and smooth

23 Apply moisturiser for the correct skin type. Follow the cleansing routine (step 9) to apply the moisturiser. Blot the skin with tissue if there is slightly too much moisturiser on the skin.

24 Leave the client to relax for a couple of minutes, and go and wash your hands. Then offer your client a mirror, so that she can check her complexion – her skin colour and its appearance.

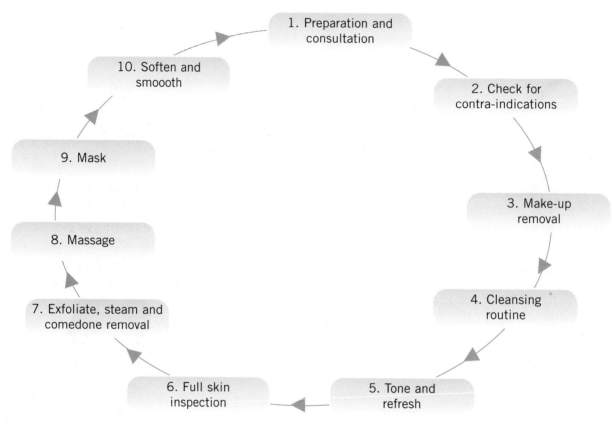

Procedure spiral for a facial treatment

> **REMEMBER**
>
> When you have finished the facial treatment, you must:
> - ask your client how she feels, and if she is pleased with her treatment
> - give your client homecare advice
> - check the finished result with the senior therapist
> - check the time, to make sure that the treatment was cost effective and carried out within an acceptable time (see Section 2 pages 67–68)
> - make sure that the workplace is left tidy, clean and ready for further treatments.

Face follow-up

The facial treatment has given your client's skin a boost. After the treatment, her skin will enjoy better circulation and a softer texture, and should be the cleanest it has been for a while. It is therefore important to give your client follow-up advice, so that she can experience the long-term benefits of her treatment. The table below details the follow-up advice that you should give.

Follow-up advice	Reasons for advice
Leave the skin alone for the next 12 hours – it is not even necessary to cleanse it that night	The skin has had an hour-long treatment to deep cleanse and stimulate it, so it is best to allow time for the skin to relax and the salon products to work
Do not apply make-up for 12 hours, if possible	Make-up could clog the skin pores and make the skin dirty again, before it has had a chance to gain the full benefits of the treatment
Avoid touching the skin	Touching the skin will make it dirty and undo the good work of the facial
Advise the client to have a monthly facial, if possible	The skin takes about a month to renew its layers, so a regular facial will keep it in great condition
Advise the client to cleanse, tone and moisturise, both morning and evening	This will keep the skin and pores clean and the skin soft
Wear a good moisturiser under make-up and in cold and windy weather	A good moisturiser will protect the skin from getting clogged with make-up and drying out in bad weather
Drink plenty of water and eat a healthy diet with lots of fruit and fresh vegetables	Water will help to re-hydrate dry skin, and a good diet will improve the condition of all skin types
Get plenty of sleep	When we sleep, the skin has a chance to repair itself
Try not to touch or squeeze blackheads and spots	You could make the problem worse and damage the skin
Always protect skin in the sun	The sun can age and dry out skin

Follow-up advice for client

Reasons why a client may not enjoy her facial

- Harming or scratching the client's skin with jewellery, watches or nails that are too long.
- Excessive or rough massage.
- Getting facial creams or products into the client's eyes.
- Breathing into the client's face.
- Not being hygienic or careful enough.
- The careless and incorrect removal of cream, for example, leaving a greasy film behind the ears or under the chin.
- Not permitting the client to relax, either by talking too much or by being tense whilst giving the treatment.

- Being disorganised, for example, leaving the room to fetch materials and products.
- If your hands are heavy, rough or cold.
- If you have offensive body odour, bad breath or tobacco smells.

 CHECK IT OUT

List five more reasons why you think a client might not enjoy her facial treatment.

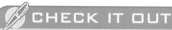 **MEMORY JOGGER**

Test yourself and see how much you can remember. You could include the answers in your portfolio.

1 Give **three** reasons why a client might want a facial.

2 List **five** contra-indications to a facial treatment.

3 The skin is made of a dead layer and a living layer. What are they called?

4 What things do you need to look for when carrying out a facial assessment?

5 List **six** things that need to be included on a client's record card.

6 Name the **three** ways in which you find out information about a client.

7 Why is it important that our workplace is set up properly? Give **six** reasons.

8 Describe briefly the following skin types:
   a dry
   b normal
   c oily
   d combination.

9 What is the purpose of:
   a cleansing
   b toning
   c moisturising?

10 List **six** face facts.

11 Explain **three** functions of the skin.

12 List **three** tech tools.

13 List **six** face basics.

14 List **three** lotions and potions.

15 Give **six** points of follow-up advice and the reasons for them.

 CHECK IT OUT

You may wish to review the chapter as revision.

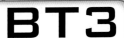
Introduction

In this unit, you will learn how to help with nail treatments and care for the hands and surrounding skin. In order to do this skilfully and confidently, you will need to show that you can:

- prepare your work area and the client for a treatment
- carry out a consultation
- carry out a basic nail treatment
- give advice.

Helping hands

Well cared for hands and nails are a great confidence booster. When a client looks down at her hands after a manicure, she will notice a big improvement, even if she cares for them well herself. A professional manicure is steps ahead of homecare, and the client should be proud to show off her hands!

 CHECK IT OUT

Look at the pictures below, showing hands before and after a manicure. Can you see a difference? Describe what you see.

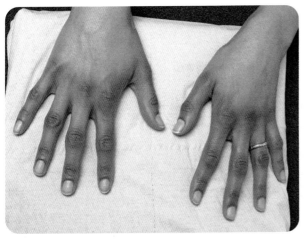

Before a manicure

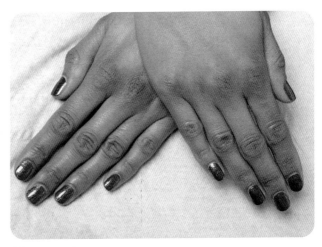

After a manicure

There are many reasons why a client may book a manicure. In addition, it is not only clients with good hands and nails who come to the salon for this treatment.

Reasons for a manicure:

❶ Brides in the weeks up to their wedding, and before the special day.

❷ Nail biters hoping that a regular manicure will help them to stop.

❸ Previous nail biters who need strengthening treatments for weak nails.

❹ For the regular upkeep of healthy nails and a well groomed appearance.

❺ To prevent tears and splits in the nail becoming more serious.

❻ Male manicures.

❼ Filing and a re-varnish, to tidy up the nails between manicures.

❽ For relaxation and a feeling of wellbeing.

❾ For specialised hand masks to treat dry cuticles and skin (not covered in Level 1).

As a beauty therapist, you will therefore need to show a lot of skill and knowledge in order to please a wide range of clients.

In this unit, you will cover the following topics:

▪ nail facts

▪ preparing to treat

▪ carry out a manicure

▪ handy tips.

Nail facts

What you will learn about:

▪ What is a manicure?
▪ Parts of the nail
▪ Functions of the parts of the nail
▪ Bones of the hand and wrist
▪ Nail health
▪ Nail shapes
▪ Fingertip facts

What is a manicure?

A manicure is a treatment carried out to improve and beautify the condition of the hands and nails. It takes about 30–45 minutes to complete and its aims are to:

▪ clean and shape the nails
▪ care for the cuticles
▪ soften dry skin on the hands
▪ relax the muscles in the hand and arm
▪ give a healthy shine to the nails.

A manicure includes:

▪ a hand and nail inspection – to check for the condition of the hands and any problem areas
▪ filing and bevelling – to neaten the nails and remove splits and catches
▪ soaking – to soften the skin for cuticle work
▪ cuticle work – to push back and neaten the cuticles
▪ massage – to moisturise the skin, improve blood flow and relax the client
▪ buffing – to smooth ridges, give a healthy shine and improve the blood flow
▪ painting – to beautify the nails by adding colour and shine.

After a manicure, the nails should look naturally polished or perfectly painted. The skin on the hands and around the cuticles should be soft and smooth.

Parts of the nail

The **nail plate** is a hard, rectangular and curved structure that covers and protects the sensitive fingertips and **nail bed**. When healthy, a nail should be pink, smooth and flexible with a white **free edge** that shows no signs of flaking or splitting. The **cuticle** should not be dry, rough or *inflamed*.

Red-looking and swollen, possibly because of an infection.

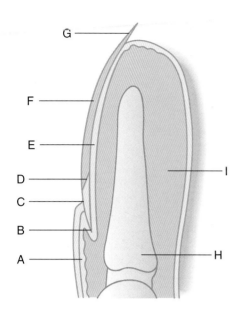

A　nail wall
B　matrix
C　cuticle
D　half moon (lanula)
E　nail bed
F　nail plate
G　free edge
H　bone
I　subcutaneous tissue

Cross-section of the nail and finger

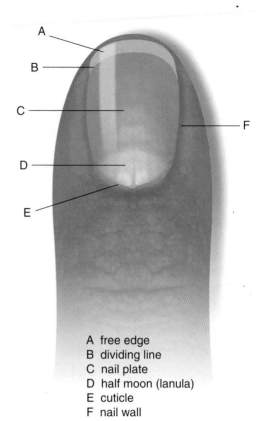

A　free edge
B　dividing line
C　nail plate
D　half moon (lanula)
E　cuticle
F　nail wall

The nail plate

Functions of the parts of the nail

The matrix

The matrix is the only living part of the nail. Its function is to grow and replace the cells that form the nail. The quality, strength and health of the nail is therefore decided in the matrix. The nail's condition depends on how healthy the cell growth is and whether or not there has been any damage to the matrix, for example, from knocks, injury (for example, a nail being shut in the door), poor treatment or an infection. However, as long as the matrix has not been permanently damaged, the effect on the nail is usually only temporary.

The lanula

The lanula is also known as the half moon. It is found on all nails, but on some it is easier to see. It is at the base of the nails and is the visible part of the matrix.

The nail bed

The nail bed is the healthy soft tissue underneath the nail plate. It gives the nail its pink appearance. It contains blood vessels and nerve endings. Ridges in the nail bed help to keep the nail firmly in place as it grows.

The nail plate

The nail plate lies on top of the nail bed and is the main part of the nail. It is pink in colour because of the soft tissue underneath, which is visible through the plate. The nail plate is made up of layers of fat, moisture and growth cells, and these give the nail its strength. If you tear part of the nail off, it is very painful because it is attached to blood vessels and nerve endings.

The free edge

The nail edge is the hardest part of the nail. It grows past the end of the nail bed and fingertip. It is whitish in colour, as it has grown beyond the pink tissue. If you break this part of the nail, it does not hurt because it is not joined to blood vessels or nerve endings.

Nail grooves or nail wall

The nail grooves are deep ridges that lie along the back and sides of the nail. The grooves at the side of the nail guide the direction of the nail growth. The grooves also help to stop germs from entering the nail bed. If the nail grooves are not kept soft and well-moisturised, *hangnails* can appear. If they are not pushed back, they can cover part of the nail plate, which makes the nail look shorter.

Dry strips of skin at the sides of the nail that can become very sore and inflamed if left untreated or pulled off.

The cuticle

The cuticle is found at the base of the nail. It is designed to protect the matrix against germs by forming a barrier. You should *never* cut the cuticle off during a manicure, as the matrix could become infected.

Bones of the hand and wrist

There are three sections to the bones of the hand and wrist. These are:

- the **carpals** in the wrist, consisting of eight bones
- the **metacarpals** in the hand or palm – there is one metacarpal on each finger and thumb
- the **phalanges** in the fingers and thumbs – there are three phalanges that make up each finger, and two phalanges on the thumb.

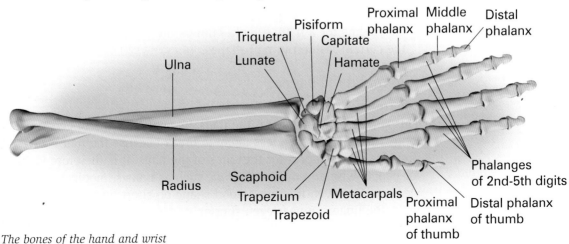

The bones of the hand and wrist

CHECK IT OUT

Take a close look at your hands. With one hand feel the bones in the other hand. See if you can make out the different bones or bone groups.

Nail health

The state of your nails can provide the secret to your health. A doctor can often tell what illness a person has by looking at the appearance of a nail. For example, some nail conditions show that a person has heart problems, poor circulation or a lack of iron.

INFORMATION

Although at Level 1, you do not need to know about this, you must *always* tell a senior therapist if you notice anything unusual when carrying out a consultation. It may be that it is not safe to carry out the nail treatment.

Nail shapes

Nail shapes vary from one client to another. The natural nail shape usually mirrors the line of the cuticle (see the different nail shapes on the next page).

When shaping nails, you need to think about:

- **the shape of the existing nail** – you cannot change the natural shape of the nail, you can only improve it.
- **the client's lifestyle and job** – for example, is she sporty or does she do manual work, in which case are long nails really practical?
- **what the client wants** – clients usually have a good idea of how they want their nails to look and what needs doing. Alternatively, they may be going somewhere special and want them painted a certain colour to match an outfit.
- **the shape of the cuticles** – when shaping the nails, follow the cuticle line for a natural look – unless the client wishes to follow the current fashion in nail shapes.

Different nail shapes

Square

This is a very good shape if the nails are short and the fingers quite long. This shape is also less likely to break because the nail wall provides good support for the sides of the nails. It is therefore ideal for people who do **manual labour**, such as typists, medical staff and cleaners. However, it is not a good shape on short fingers, as it can make the fingers appear even shorter.

Work involving the hands.

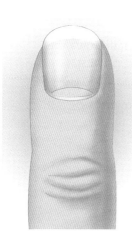
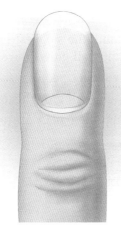
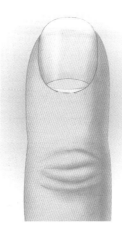
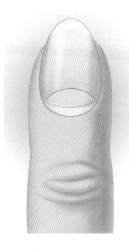

Square   *Oval*   *Round*   *Pointed*

Oval

This all-purpose nail shape flatters and softens the appearance of the hands. It makes the fingers look longer. It is also quite hardwearing against breakage, because of its smooth edges and flexible shape.

Round

This is also a very practical nail shape. It is hardwearing, strong and neat. However, it is not very flattering as it doesn't help to make the fingers look longer.

Pointed

Some clients prefer this nail shape, as they believe it makes their nails look longer. However, it is best to advise against this shape, as the nails are filed to a point from the corners to the tip. The corners where the free edge starts are the **stress points** of the nails – the nails have no support from the nail wall so can easily weaken and split.

The parts where the nail is weakest.

Fingertip facts

1. The nails are held together with fats and moisture; you can peel back one or two layers when the nails are out of condition.
2. Nails dry out as we get older.
3. The ridges on a nail are natural and are there to help the nail plate stick to the nail bed. If the nails are filed or buffed to get a smooth look, this will weaken the nail. However, very deep ridges can be a sign of illness.
4. Fingernails take 3–6 months to grow from root to tip.
5. Toenails take 10–12 months to grow from root to tip.
6. On average, nails grow one eighth of an inch (0.3 cm) per month.
7. Nails grow faster in the summer than in the winter.
8. If a person is right-handed, his or her fingernails will grow faster on the right hand than on the left hand. This is because the person's right hand gets more stimulation. (The reverse is true for left-handed people.)

> **CHECK IT OUT**
>
> Look at the different nail shapes on your fellow students. Which are the most common?

9 Men's nails grow faster than women's nails.

10 The longer the finger, the faster the nail growth.

11 Of the nails on the hand, the smallest finger nail grows the slowest, and the thumb nail grows the second slowest.

12 Nails grow faster in younger people.

13 If we diet too much, our nail growth slows down.

14 If left to grow too long, the nails start to curl.

If left to grow too long, nails curl

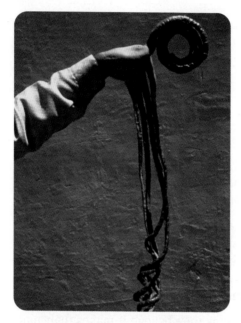

Prepare to Treat

What you will learn about:

- In your hands
- Client consultation
- Lotions and potions
- The workspace
- Nail basics
- Tech tools

In your hands

 CHECK IT OUT

Briefly describe how you think your hands and nails should look when giving a treatment, so that a client will not be put off, but will feel confident that she is being treated by a person who knows what she is doing.

THINK ABOUT IT

Think about your self-preparation. You will be assisting with a nail treatment, so how do you think your hands and nails should look? Should they be dirty, bitten and rough with chipped varnish? Should they be uneven lengths or too long?

The workspace
Where and how?

A manicure can be carried out in a variety of ways, and some of these are better than others are.

- Some salons have an area especially set up for manicures, with good lighting and all equipment and products at hand. This is the best practice for manicure treatments.

- In other salons, a manicure is carried out in the reception area or as an extra part of a treatment. This is not best practice, and can be awkward for both the client and the therapist.

Ways that a manicure can be carried out are:

- **across a couch** – with the client on one side and you on the other, and the products laid out next to you.

- **at a manicure station** – this is a trolley on wheels designed especially for carrying out manicures. It usually has drawers for storage and sometimes has a magnifying lamp. There should be room for the client to sit one side of the station, and for the therapist to sit on the other side.

- **the client sits in a couch or chair while the therapist sits on a manicure stool.** The manicure stool has a cushioned seat, a swinging arm for resting and supporting the client's hands and arms, and drawers underneath for the storage of products.

- **the therapist sits to the side of a client while she is having her hair done.** This is a very unsatisfactory way of carrying out a manicure. It is difficult for the therapist to carry out the manicure in comfort, which could affect the standard of the manicure.

- **the therapist sits to the side of the treatment couch while the client has a facial.** Again, this is not the best way to carry out a manicure. Either the client will have to stretch one of her arms across her body, or the therapist will have to swap sides to carry out the treatment on the second hand.

REMEMBER

When you set up, make sure that the tools and equipment are positioned so that you don't have to bend over to reach them. If you are right-handed, position the tools and equipment on the left. If you are left-handed, position them on the right. This helps to prevent you from knocking things over.

This may seem obvious, but when you are busy remembering other things, this could easily be overlooked.

Posture and lighting

Posture
Since manicures are the only treatment that can be organised in so many different ways, and can take place in so many different locations, it is especially important that you pay attention to your posture. Whichever method and whatever location your salon uses for manicures, it is important that you make sure that both you and your client are comfortable. If your back is overstretched from reaching when carrying out the treatment, it will cause you back pain, neck ache and tiredness.

Therefore, once you have decided where you will be carrying out your manicure, you must make sure that:

■ you and your client are not too cramped – there should be plenty of room for both of you to move your arms and legs freely

■ the client is not positioned too far from you. You must be able to reach her hands and arms without having to lean over or stretch up.

Lighting

In order to see the nail plate, cuticles and polish during a manicure, good overhead or natural lighting is essential. When carrying out a manicure, you should always check the following.

■ Is the light bright enough?

■ Does the light cast shadows?

These may be a particular problem if you are positioned in the corner of a room.

Health and hygiene

The differences between sanitisation, disinfection and sterilisation were covered in Section 2 (pages 28–29). Let's now think about the practical side of health and hygiene for manicures and pedicures. The table below shows how and why cross-infection can occur.

THINK ABOUT IT

If a manicure is carried out during a facial, when the light has been dimmed to help relaxation, would this be good practice? Why?

Potential cross-infection during a nail treatment

Manicure and pedicure	What could happen	How infections could start
The therapist has not washed her hands before the treatment	Illness and skin infections	The therapist goes to the toilet and then continues the treatment
		The therapist has handled money before starting the treatment (money is covered in many germs)
		The therapist has completed a treatment on one client and then carried straight on to the next client
Soaking nails in water	Veruccas and other conditions	Using water that has previously been used on a client with a *verucca*
		Bits of skin floating in the water, either from the soles of the feet or the fingernails, which contain germs and dirt
Pushing back cuticles	Swollen and infected cuticles	Cuticle tools that have not been sterilised and are covered in germs, which are then used on different clients
Moisturising hands and feet	Skin infections	The therapist uses her fingers to scoop out the cream from the pot instead of a disposable spatula. After a few treatments, the cream is full of germs from different clients

A wart on the foot.

REMEMBER

The results of cross-infection are horrible, so make sure that you always follow the correct hygiene methods when giving a treatment. The results of not being hygienic could be very damaging for both the salon and your career.

Client consultation

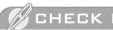 **CHECK IT OUT**

Review Section 3: Treatment Essentials (pages 75–76)

You are now going to look at the information you need to find out from a client before carrying out a manicure consultation.

You will watch a senior therapist carrying out a consultation at first and eventually, as you gain experience, you will be able to carry out a consultation yourself under supervision. Watch and listen carefully.

Name

It is best to have a record of both the client's first name and surname. It is important to record the first name because there could be two clients with the same surname. If you only write the surname, this could cause confusion and client records may become mixed up.

Address

Write the client's full address including postcode.

Telephone number

Always write down a home number and a work or mobile number. One telephone number is not enough – if a client's appointment needs to be cancelled at short notice, you will not be able to contact her if she is at work and you only have her home telephone number!

The client's lifestyle and job

This information will help you to understand how much the client uses her hands. This will tell you whether she is able to grow her nails long or needs to keep them short.

The client's reason for the manicure and her needs/wishes for today

Asking this information of your client will help you to understand what she needs from her manicure treatment. For example, does she want her nails manicured and painted for a special occasion, or is this a treatment simply to keep her nails neat and tidy?

Condition of hands/nails when inspected

When you carry out a consultation, you will need to find out information from your client to help you build a picture of what she needs from her nail treatment. You will need to do this by:

▪ **Questioning**

This is when you ask the client questions about her hands, nails and wishes for the treatment.

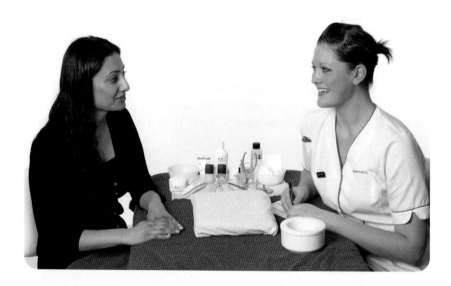

Questioning a client before a manicure

▪ **Visual inspection**

This is when you look at the client's hands, nails, skin colour and texture.

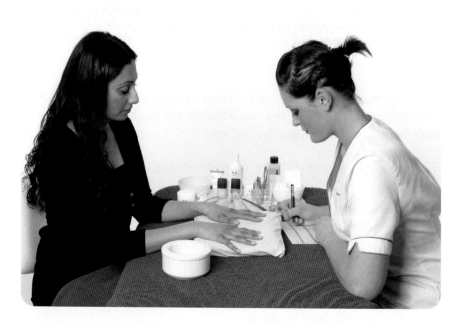

Performing a visual inspection before a manicure

Manual inspection

This is when you feel the client's skin on her hands, and her cuticles and nails.

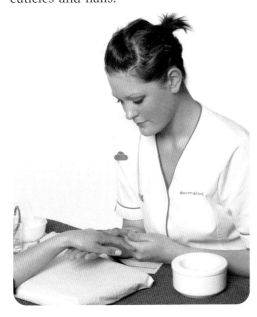

Carrying out a manual inspection before a manicure

Assessing the condition

When inspecting the hands, make notes under the following headings:

- **Hands**
  - Examine the front and the backs of the hands.
  - Look at the colour and texture of the skin – is it tanned or pale? Is the skin thin or thickened?
  - Are the hands soft and smooth, or are they rough and chapped?
  - Does the skin show any signs of infection, such as swelling, pus or lifting of the nail plate? Are there cracks and breaks in the skin, or redness around the cuticles?
  - Look at the skin between the fingers – are there any signs of dryness?

- **Nails**
  - What shape are the nails?
  - What length are the nails? Are they long or short? Have they been bitten?
  - Are the nails healthy – strong, pink, shiny and flexible? Are they unhealthy – yellow, brittle, weak and thin?
  - Do the nails show any signs of nail diseases or disorders?

- **Skin around the nails**
  - Are the cuticles hard and overgrown, red and inflamed, or smooth and even?
  - Have the cuticles grown along the nail plate?
  - Are there any hangnails?

Contra-indications and conditions

Are there any signs of nail or hand disorders or infections? If yes, then:

- can they be worked around if covered?
- are they a total contra-indication?
- will you be able to treat the client if she has her doctor's permission?

Manicure contra-indications and conditions

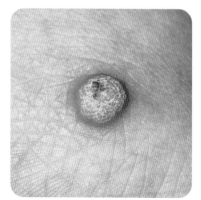

Warts

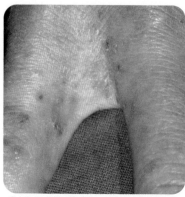

Scabies

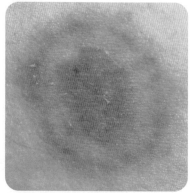

Ringworm

Grazes and scratches.

Redness and possibly swelling.

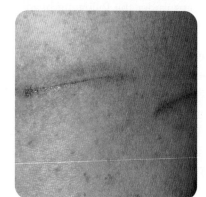

*Cuts and **abrasions***

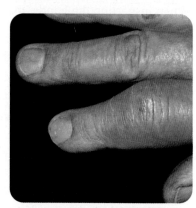

*Swelling and **inflammation***

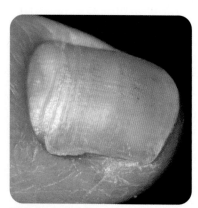

Discoloured nails

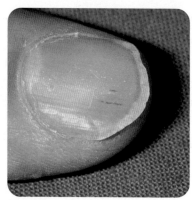

Damaged nails

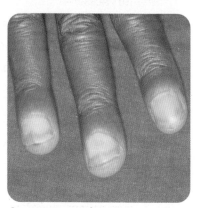

Overgrown cuticles

Products used

In addition to the everyday products used in a manicure, did you use extras such as nail strengtheners and ridge fillers? Here, you should also list the varnish colour you used, in case the client wants the same colour next time.

Homecare advice

What advice did you give your client on how she could improve the condition of her hands and nails? When did you advise her to return for another salon treatment?

MANICURE/PEDICURE CONSULTATION SHEET

DATE _20/3/04_   NAME _Jon Bomero_

ADDRESS _Flat c, Westbrook, St Giles Road, Tonmouth_

TELEPHONE NUMBER (H) _(01121) 556600_   (W) _(01121) 818120_

CONDITION OF HANDS/NAILS ON INSPECTION

Hands - dry and chapped

Nails - cuticles dry and overgrown. Nails thick and stong

CONTRA-INDICATIONS

None

PRODUCTS USED

Simply Men manicure range

PRODUCT SALES

HOMECARE ADVICE

Carry out a salt and oil rub to help remove dry skin but avoid any

chapped areas. Use moisturiser daily.

COMMENTS

Removed excess cuticles, buffed nails.

Advised client to return monthly.

RECORD OF TREATMENTS

DATE	TREATMENT	THERAPIST
13/1/03	manicure	S Jones
20/3/04	manicure	Nadia Hoffman

A typical consultation card for a manicure or pedicure treatment

Product sales

Did you sell the client any products or nail varnishes, or advise her to buy them in the future?

Record of treatments

Write the date, the type of manicure, the therapist's name and any extra notes that could be useful for the future.

Comments

What were the results of the manicure? Any advice to other therapists? Here, you should write whatever you think may be useful to you or another therapist in the future.

 SALON STORY

During a consultation with her client, Eve realised that what the client wanted was not in her best interests. The client's nails were dry and brittle, and the cuticles were very hard and slightly inflamed with skin that had grown along the nail plate. The client wanted a basic manicure and her nails painted a bright red colour – she had brought the colour in herself.

Eve very politely set about advising her client that, rather than a basic manicure, her nails needed some tender care. She advised a six-week course of intensive moisturising and nourishing treatments to get the cuticles and nails back into good condition.

What homecare advice should Eve provide to the client to get her nails back into good condition?

Nail basics

Cotton wool

To remove nail varnish, the cotton wool is rolled into small balls and each ball is soaked with nail varnish remover. A clean piece of cotton wool is used for each nail.

Cotton wool is also used to cover the tip of an orange stick, for cuticle work, the application of cream and nail cleaning.

Tissues

Tissues are used for various things during a manicure, for example, wiping products from the nail. As mentioned on page 104, 1-ply split tissues are used rather than 2-ply tissues.

Towels

A towel is used to dry the hands and fingers of
the client after they have been soaked in water
during a manicure. Towels are also used to
protect a client's clothing if she is not wearing
a gown.

Gown

The client wears a gown to protect her clothing
from spills or splashes of a product.

Dishes

Small plastic or metal dishes are needed to hold
cotton wool and tissues, as well as the client's
jewellery. Any jewellery left on during the
manicure will get in the way of the treatment
and become coated in hand cream.

Waste bin or container

A pedal bin with a lid is best for hygiene
purposes, as you can open it without touching it
with your hands. However, if you are doing a
manicure in a corner of a room or an area
without a pedal bin, then you can use a waste
paper bin lined with a disposable bag. After the
treatment, make sure that the bin is emptied,
and the bag is sealed and placed in a waste bin with a lid.

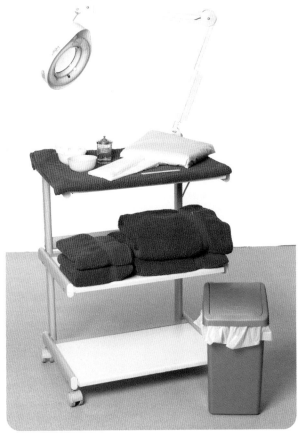

Nail basics

If a bowl or container other than a bin is used for waste, make sure
that you have lined it with couch roll first. This will allow you to
scoop the waste up easily after the treatment. Remember to wash and
disinfect the bowl afterwards.

Sterilising jar

This should be filled with antiseptic or disinfectant solution, so that
small metal tools that have been previously sterilised can be placed in
it during the treatment. The solution will help to keep germ levels
down, but it will not destroy germs completely. The solution should
be changed after every client.

Manicure cushion

These provide extra comfort during the manicure. They allow the
client to rest her hands and also give support to the wrist.

Manicure cushions usually have a removable washable cover made
from towelling. However, if the cushion does not have a cover, then a
protective towel should be placed on top.

Manicure bowl

This is a specially shaped gripper bowl, which has a small hole in it for the thumb and a larger hole for the rest of the fingers. It is filled with warm soapy water to soak the client's hands during the manicure. It has a removable lid so that it can be cleaned thoroughly inside after each treatment.

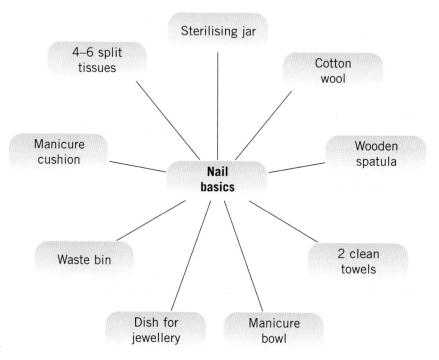

Nail basics for manicure treatment

Lotions and potions

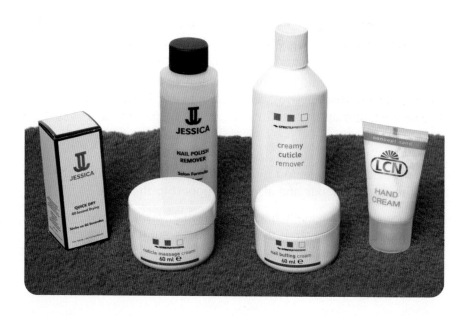

Nail lotions and potions

Nail varnish remover

This dissolves nail varnish so that it can be wiped off the nail plate easily with a piece of cotton wool. Nail varnish remover has a drying effect on the nail, so it usually contains a small amount of oil to moisturise the nail.

Cuticle cream

This is a thick moisturising cream that is used to soften and nourish the cuticle, so that the cuticle can be pushed back more easily during a manicure, without the skin splitting or pulling.

Cuticle remover

This is a milky-coloured liquid that contains an active ingredient to dissolve skin cells. It is used to loosen any cuticle that sticks to and grows along the nail plate. It also acts as a nail shampoo, because it contains an active ingredient to bleach out stains. The senior therapist will demonstrate and carry out this part of the nail treatment.

INFORMATION

Cuticle remover *must* be removed from the skin completely, immediately after use. This is because it can carry on dissolving the skin cells, which could make the skin very sore, dry and irritated.

Buffing paste

Buffing paste contains an **abrasive ingredient** that is used to smooth out fine ridges on the surface of the nail. It also helps to remove surface stains on the nail plate. Buffing paste leaves the nails with a shiny surface and can be used instead of nail varnish.

A rough and scratchy substance that is used to clean a smooth surface.

Moisturiser or massage cream

This is a rich cream that is massaged into the hands and arms at the end of the manicure and before the nail painting.

Nail varnish dryer

A nail varnish dryer doesn't dry the nails completely, however, it helps them to harden more quickly. It comes in the form of a spray or 'paint on' product (similar to clear nail varnish), and can be oil or alcohol based.

INFORMATION

After painting the nails, the natural hardening time can be up to two hours. Even if the nails feel dry to touch, they can still dent if they are knocked, so it is best to advise the client not to dig into her handbag for her keys!

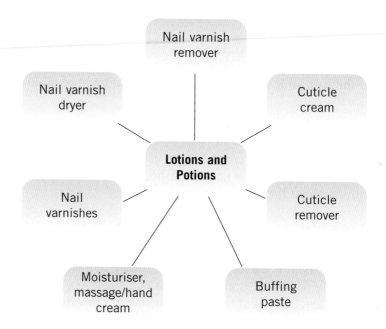

Nail varnish remover

Nail varnish dryer

Cuticle cream

Lotions and Potions

Nail varnishes

Cuticle remover

Moisturiser, massage/hand cream

Buffing paste

Nail lotions and potions

Tech tools

Spatula

A spatula is used for scooping out products hygienically.

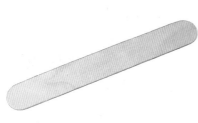

Spatula

Emery board

This is a thin card file with an abrasive covering on each side. It is used for filing and shaping the nails. The fine side is used for fingernails and the coarse side for male manicures and toenails, as they tend to be thicker than the fingernails. Emery boards come in different sizes and widths, and some have funky designs on them. They should be disposed of after use, for hygiene purposes.

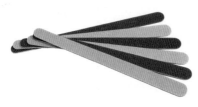

Emery board

Orange sticks

These are made of orange wood, which is slightly bendy. One end is pointed and the other end is shaped like a hoof. Both ends of the orange stick are coated in cotton wool for hygiene purposes, as the cotton wool can be removed and thrown away after use. The cotton wool also softens the tip, which prevents the cuticles and skin becoming sore during treatment. The pointed end is used for cleaning under the free edge of the nail, and the hoof end is used for cuticle work.

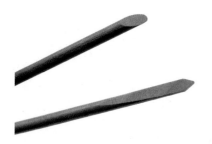

Orange stick

INFORMATION

Emery boards and orange sticks don't cost much to the salon, and as they are difficult to sterilise it is a good idea to give them to the client at the end of her manicure, as an extra bonus. She will leave happy and pampered from the treatment, and grateful for the small gift.

Rubber hoof stick

In addition to the orange stick, this tool can also be used to push back the cuticles safely. At the end of the wooden stick is a hoof-shaped rubber piece. However, once it has been sterilised a few times, the rubber tends to fall apart, so the hoof stick needs to be replaced regularly.

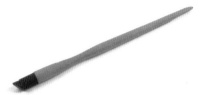

Rubber hoof stick

Nail brush

This can be used during the nail soaking, to gently rub away staining around the fingers or on the nails. It is also used to remove cuticle remover. However, it is not a very hygienic tool as it is extremely difficult to sterilise completely and can harbour germs in-between the bristles.

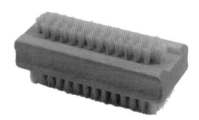

Nail brush

Nail buffer

This is made of chamois and used with a buffing paste to shine the nail plate. The action of the buffing also improves the blood flow to the nails, which encourages nail growth.

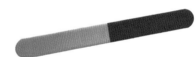

Nail buffer

Nail scissors

These are curved scissors that can be used to cut long nails before filing – when it would take too long to use an emery board.

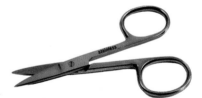

INFORMATION

When cutting nails, the nail plate must be held firmly and supported so that the cutting action doesn't hurt or cause damage to the layers of the nail.

Curved nail scissors

Cuticle knife

This blunt, straight-edged tool is used to gently free any cuticle that has stuck to the nail plate. This is done by applying light pressure and making small circular movements at the base of the nail. When using this tool, you should be careful not to use a digging and pushing-back action, as this will only damage the matrix and make the cuticles sore. However, this tool is not used at Level 1.

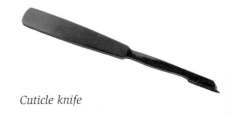

Cuticle knife

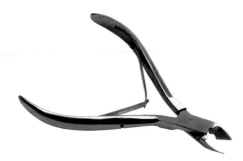

Cuticle nippers

Cuticle nippers

These cutting tools do *not* cut the main part of the cuticles, as the name suggests. Instead, they are used gently to cut away extra skin that has grown down the nail from dry, uncared-for cuticles. They are used *only* after the cuticle has been softened and loosened with cuticle remover and a hoof stick or cuticle knife. However, this tool is not used at Level 1.

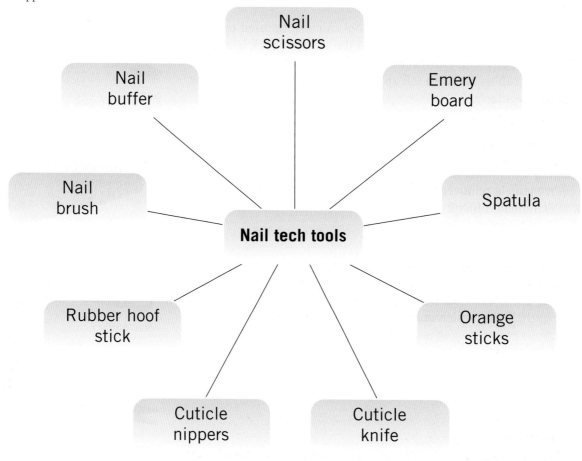

Nail tech tools

 CHECK IT OUT

How many nail basics, lotions and potions, and tech tools can you remember? In pairs, look at each list for one minute. Then test each other's memory.

Carry out a manicure

What you will learn about:

- Before you start
- Sanitising and nail varnish removal
- Filing and cuticle work
- Massage and moisturise
- Paint and polish
- Fingernail follow-up

Before you start

Before you begin the nail manicure treatment, you should:

- make a quick check of your workplace preparation
- wash your hands
- remove both your own and your client's watch and jewellery
- protect the client's clothing
- carry out a consultation
- assess the condition of your client's hands and nails
- check for contra-indications.

 REMEMBER

Explain to your client what you are doing as you go along and why, because it is important to keep the client *informed*. Chat to the client about her wishes for today's treatment. Remember that these can change from one week to the next, so remember to check each time.

Aware of what is going on.

INFORMATION

It helps to have a checklist of the tech tools, lotions and potions, and nail basics on a record card that you can keep nearby, for reference. Cover the list with a plastic cover so that it doesn't get marked, or have it laminated so that you can wipe it clean.

 REMEMBER

Always ask a senior member of staff to double check that you have not overlooked any infection or problem.

Sanitising and nail varnish removal

REMEMBER

A fresh piece of cotton wool should be used for each nail, because once there is a build-up of dissolved varnish on the cotton wool ball, it is not as good at removing varnish.

Filing and cuticle work
The right way to file nails

Do not saw in both directions, as this will cause the nail to split. Use the file at a 45-degree angle to the nail and file from one side of the nail to the centre, then file from the other side of the nail to the centre.

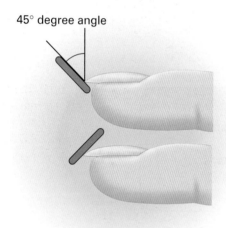

45° degree angle

45-degree angle to nail

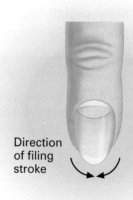

Direction of filing stroke

Side to centre action

INFORMATION

If the nails are very long and need cutting, this is best done after they have been softened by soaking in water (step 8). Cutting hard, dry nails will cause the nail layers to separate and the nails to split.

REMEMBER

Cuticle cream both softens the cuticles so that they are easier to push back, and moisturises dry skin and nails. Don't be wasteful! Any leftover cream can be used for the other hand.

STEP-BY-STEP MANICURE 1

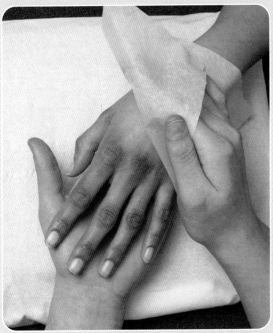

1 Wipe over the front and back of both of your client's hands with antiseptic

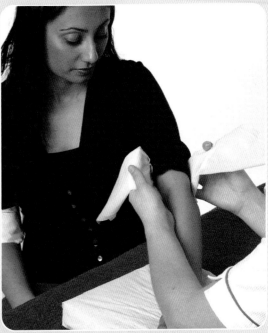

2 Roll your client's sleeves up to the elbow, then tuck tissue around them for protection against creams and lotions

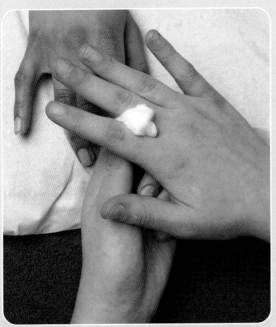

3 Right hand. Soak a clean ball of cotton wool with nail varnish remover, then place between two fingers. Hold onto the nail plate for a few seconds, then wipe downwards to remove the dissolved varnish

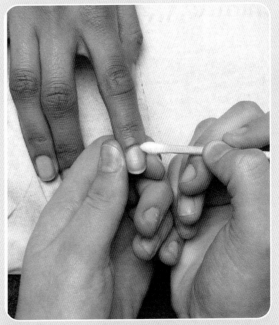

4 Right hand. Cover an orange stick with cotton wool, then dip the end into some nail varnish remover. Use this to go round the cuticle and nail fold, where bright varnish tends to stain

STEP-BY-STEP MANICURE 2

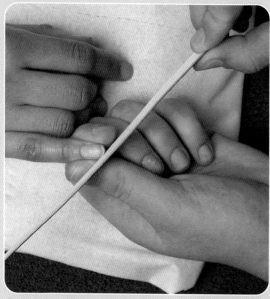

5 File the nails on the right hand using the fine side of the emery board

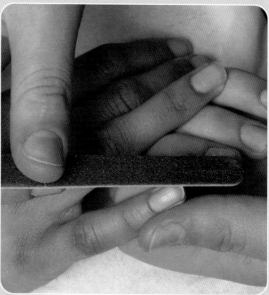

6 Right hand. Turn the emery board lengthways to the nail and very gently buff the tip of the nail with the fine side. This action is called bevelling. Bevelling seals the free edges of the nail, and this prevents them from splitting and peeling back

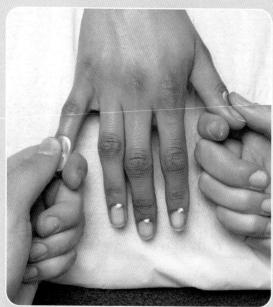

7 Right hand. Use a clean spatula to scoop out a small (pea-sized) amount of cuticle cream. Next, dip a covered orange stick into the cream and apply it to the centre of the cuticles on each nail. Massage in the cuticle cream in a circular action, so that it covers the nail and cuticles

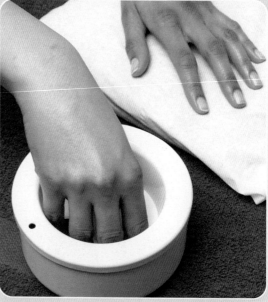

8 Place your client's right hand in the gripper bowl containing warm soapy water. On the client's left hand, repeat steps 3–8

STEP-BY-STEP MANICURE 3

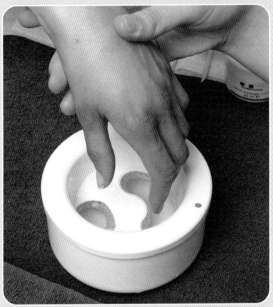

9 Take your client's right hand out of the water. Place the client's left hand in the water

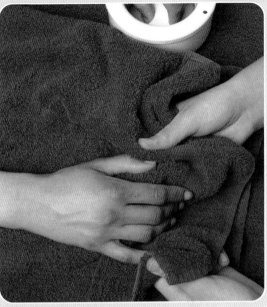

10 Dry the client's right hand and nails thoroughly using a towel, pushing the cuticles back with the towel as you go

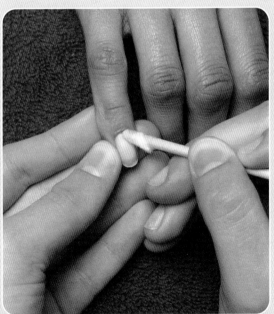

11 On the right hand, the senior therapist uses a clean covered orange stick to apply cuticle remover (that has been placed on a spatula) to the cuticles of each nail and underneath the free edge. With the orange stick, push back gently using circular actions, and clean under the free edge

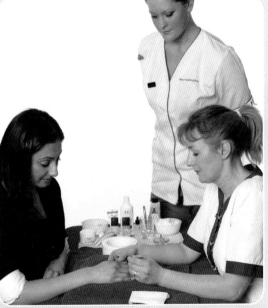

12 The senior therapist may need to ease away any excess cuticle with a cuticle knife. If there are any hangnails or loose bits of skin on the cuticles she will also need to use the cuticle nippers to remove them.

REMEMBER

Cuticle remover acts as a nail shampoo and will help get rid of staining or stubborn dirt. Place any loose bits of cuticle or dirt on a tissue and throw away afterwards.

REMEMBER

Cuticle remover must be wiped off thoroughly, otherwise it may carry on working and could cause soreness.

INFORMATION

Scarf nail is the name for fine wisps of nail that stick out after soaking. They are very flimsy and thin, like a scarf.

Massage and moisturise

Moisturising softens and smoothes the skin and is a perfect finish to a manicure. The moisturiser or massage cream is applied and rubbed into the skin using rubbing and kneading movements (see page 152).

INFORMATION

For Level 1, it is not necessary for you to follow a set massage routine using all the movements. However, it is important that you carry out some sort of massage routine that is relaxing to the client.

A simple massage routine is to start with lighter strokes that become deeper. Begin with the arm up to the elbow, then move down to the hands and the fingers. The hand and arm massage routine should take about 5–10 minutes to complete on both hands.

 REMEMBER

After you have carried out a massage using a rich moisturising or massage cream (steps 17–20) there may still be some cream on the nail. If it remains on the nail, the nail varnish will not go on smoothly and will not dry properly. If you do manage to paint nail varnish on the nails, the varnish will soon peel off once you have finished. It is therefore very important that you de-grease the nails thoroughly with nail varnish remover.

STEP-BY-STEP MANICURE 4

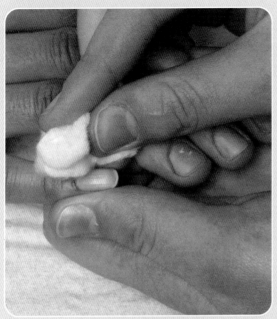

13 Remove the last traces of cuticle remover with a damp piece of cotton wool. Throw away the used cotton wool

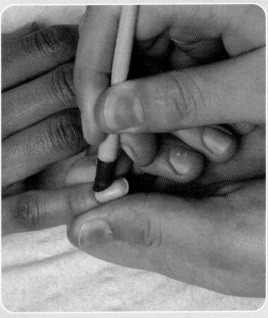

14 Finally push back treated cuticle with a rubber hoof stick

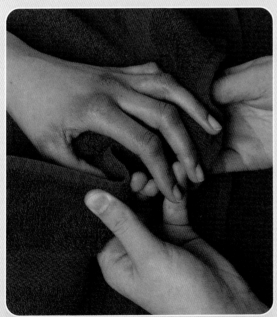

15 Take the client's left hand out of the water. Dry the client's left hand and nails thoroughly using a towel, pushing the cuticles back with the towel as you go. Repeat steps 11–15 on the client's left hand

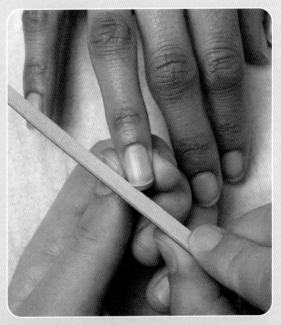

16 Tidy up the free edges of the nails on both hands with the emery board, because very fine wisps of nail may have appeared, called scarf nail

STEP-BY-STEP MANICURE 5

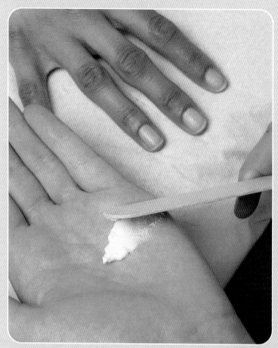

17 Using a spatula, place a small amount of massage cream or hand cream into the palm of your hands

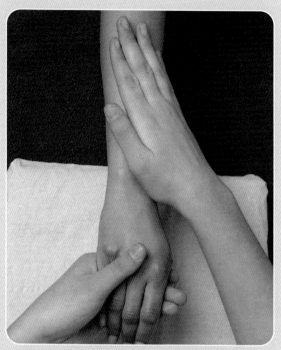

18 Stroke the cream onto the skin of your client's arms using smooth upward effleurage movements

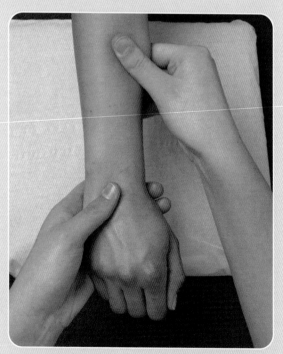

19 Massage using a variety of flowing effleurage and gentle kneading (petrissage) movements

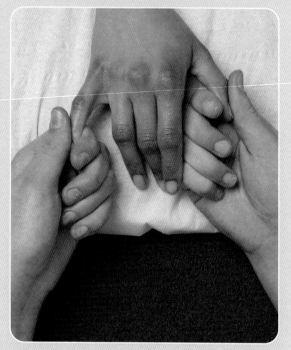

20 Finally, use petrissage techniques on the fingers of both hands. Hand massage should take about 5 minutes

STEP-BY-STEP MANICURE 6

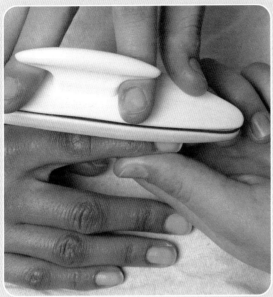

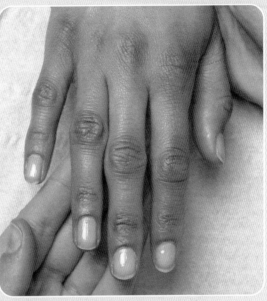

㉑ Apply a small dot of buffing paste to the centre of each nail. Quickly smooth out the dots with your thumbs. Stroke the buffer down the nail, from the base to the free edge, using a light quick movement

㉒ After you have finished buffing, your client's nails should have a healthy, natural shine. If your client prefers to have nail varnish applied, show her the colour range and ask her to choose a colour

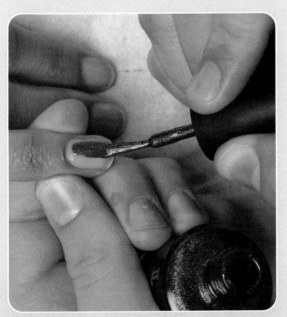

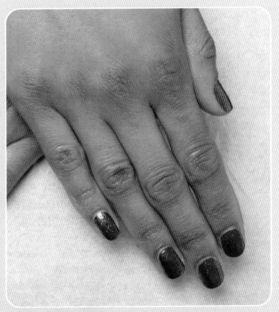

㉓ Go over the nail with nail varnish remover to de-grease, as you did at the start of your manicure (step 3). Paint the nails, following the routine described (on pages 154–55)

㉔ Check the finished result – the paint or polish completes the look

Paint and polish
Buffing

If a client chooses not to have her nails painted, offer to buff them for her. This will improve the circulation in her nails and polish them, leaving a healthy, natural shine.

> **INFORMATION**
>
> Do not rub while buffing as this will create heat, which can be painful as well as damaging to the layers of the nail. Do about four to six strokes on each nail in a downward direction. Do not be tempted to do any more strokes.

Painting

> **INFORMATION**
>
> If the client wants a varnish, now is the time to ask her to put all her jewellery back on, to put on her jacket or coat, and to get her car keys out of her handbag. You should also politely ask if she would like to pay for the manicure before you paint her nails, explaining about the drying time of varnishes. Do not demand the money!

Careful and organised, paying attention to detail.

Nail varnish should be painted on in a **methodical** way. Below are diagrams to show you how best to do this.

Painting your client's nails:

1. Make sure that your client's nails are 'squeaky' clean – there should be no dirt or grease on them.
2. Prepare a cotton wool coated orange stick by soaking it in nail vanish remover. This is in case you make a mistake while painting or to clean off any varnish around the cuticle. It is better to remove the nail varnish straight away, because wet nail varnish is easier to remove than dry nail varnish.
3. Paint the nails. While painting, support the client's hand while holding the nail varnish bottle and complete the strokes with your other hand.

When painting the nails, begin with one central application (1), then apply the varnish to the right (2) and the left (3) of the nail. Finally, go over the whole nail to smooth the varnish (4)

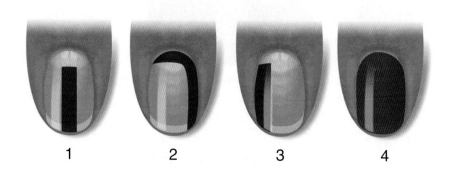

1   2   3   4

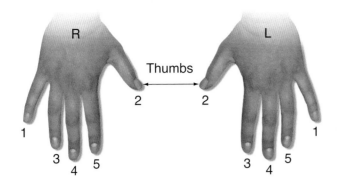

To prevent smudging, follow the finger rotation method

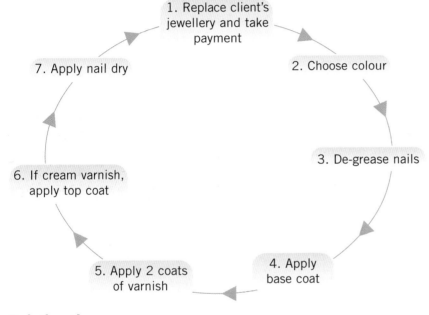

1. Replace client's jewellery and take payment
2. Choose colour
3. De-grease nails
4. Apply base coat
5. Apply 2 coats of varnish
6. If cream varnish, apply top coat
7. Apply nail dry

Procedure spiral for painting nails

Painting tips

Do:

- make sure that you have enough varnish on the brush to do the whole nail
- paint thinly
- use only a few strokes
- leave a small gap at the base of the nail before the cuticle
- hold the bottle while you paint.

Don't:

- overload the brush with paint, as it will drip down and flood the nail with too much varnish
- paint thickly, as it will take too long to dry
- use too many brush strokes, as the finish will be lumpy and uneven
- paint right up to the cuticle, as the varnish will seep into the skin and will look messy
- dip the brush in a bottle that is not held, as it could fall over and spill varnish.

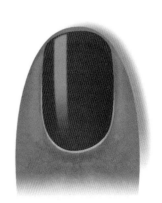

While painting, leave a small gap at the base of the nail before the cuticle

Polish profile

Base coats
These can be clear or pale coloured. They are applied to the nail plate before varnish to:

- smooth the nail
- to cut down on staining from bright coloured varnishes
- help prevent early chipping or wearing off of the colour.

Top coats
These are usually clear and are used to:

- give a high shine to the coloured nails
- help to make the varnish last longer.

Some top coats also have an added ingredient which helps to speed up the drying time.

INFORMATION

Base coats and top coats can be used if a client wants a clear varnish instead of a colour varnish.

Ridge filling base coats
These are usually pale in colour and thicker than normal base coats. If a client has a very uneven nail plate with ridges or dips, the ridge filler will help to smooth the surface of the nail.

Nail hardeners
These are clear varnishes but have ingredients that are meant to provide the nails with a tough coating

Nail strengtheners
These are usually clear and have nourishing and strengthening ingredients to help weak nails grow.

Cream nail varnish
Cream nail varnish is better for nails with many ridges and dents, as it doesn't show them up. The basic rule with cream nail varnish is:

- base coat
- two coats of cream varnish
- top coat.

Pearlised nail varnish
Pearlised nail varnish contains ingredients that give it a shimmery look. However, it shows up uneven surfaces in the nail plate, so should not be used on nails that are not healthy looking and smooth. With pearlised varnishes, the basic rule is:

- base coat
- 2–3 coats of varnish
- *No* top coat.

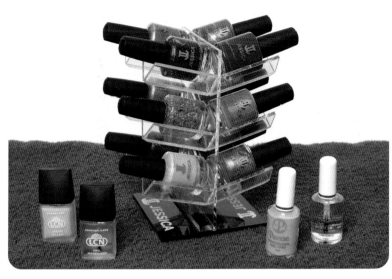

Nail polish products

Solvents

Although not a varnish product, solvents are used to dissolve nail varnishes from furniture and clothes if they have been spilled, although this process isn't always completely successful. However, the main use of solvent is to thin out nail varnishes when they become thick and sticky. A few drops in a bottle of varnish when shaken gives new life to a varnish, leaving it as thin as when it was first used.

Choosing a nail varnish colour

Nail varnish comes in many colours. As a beauty therapist, you need to be aware of a few things before you can help your client choose the best nail varnish colour.

The length of the nails

Very bright colours on short or bitten nails will only draw attention to them and make the nails look shorter than they are.

The condition of the cuticles

Red-looking cuticles can look worse if the nails are painted in a bright or pearlised varnish. Pale and neutral colours in a cream varnish look better.

The client's home life and job

If a client has a job that could cause the nails to chip quite quickly, then it is best to have a colour that is not going to show the odd little chip too much.

The client's skin colour

Orange, peach or beige colours show up the bluish colour in skin with poor circulation. Pinks clash with reddish skin tones.

The condition and smoothness of the nails

Pearlised varnish will show up any imperfections, such as dents and ridges, so use a ridge filling base coat and a cream varnish.

The size of the fingernails

Dark colours make the nails look smaller.

INFORMATION

The whole manicure treatment should take about 45 minutes. However, it may take longer until you are familiar with the routine. A handy tip is to use the manicure spiral below as a checklist and a reminder of the next stage in the treatment.

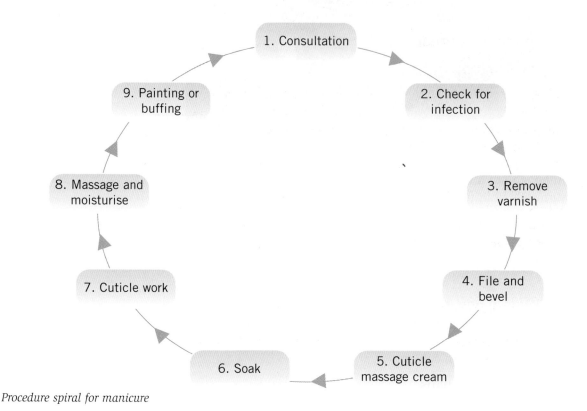

1. Consultation
2. Check for infection
3. Remove varnish
4. File and bevel
5. Cuticle massage cream
6. Soak
7. Cuticle work
8. Massage and moisturise
9. Painting or buffing

Procedure spiral for manicure

Fingernail follow-up

After the manicure, you should advise your client on how best to look after her nails so that they remain in the best condition.

Homecare advice for clients

1. Wear rubber gloves when washing up or using strong cleaning products.
2. Keep hand cream by the sink and apply it after washing up. Wear hand cream at night.
3. Wear gardening gloves – don't use bare hands in the garden.
4. Don't use your nails as tools, as this will weaken or break them.
5. Rinse off harsh products from the skin immediately, as they could cause a rash or soreness.
6. Remove rings before washing, so that soap does not build up under the rings and irritate the skin.
7. If there is a split on the nail, bevel it gently as soon as possible. (You may have to show your client what to do.)

8 Keep an emery board with you at all times, so that you can smooth away any catch in the nail instantly.

9 Apply a top coat of polish over painted nails every other day, to make the varnish last longer.

10 Don't be tempted to pick dry cuticles – use a rich cream to soften them.

11 Always use a base coat under varnish to protect the nails from becoming stained.

12 Try to make time for a manicure every two weeks.

Complete the treatment

When the whole manicure and painting treatment is complete, you will need to check that the client is happy with the result. The easiest and most obvious way is to ask her. If there is anything that she is not happy about, then it is your job to put it right with the help of your supervisor.

If the client is satisfied with her treatment, you will then need to check that the finished effect meets the senior therapist's approval and that you completed the treatment within a commercially viable time (see Section 2, pages 67–68).

REMEMBER

Leaving your work area clean and tidy ready for the next treatment is essential. Replace all furniture, put away products, replace dirty laundry, wipe surfaces, re-sterilise tools and get clean disinfectant.

INFORMATION

If the client is happy with her manicure and likes the products that you have used, it would be a good idea to ask her if she would like to look at the products on sale. Handy take-home packs are a good selling point, as they allow the client to continue with her nail care at home.

Handy tips

What you will learn about:

- No more chips
- Tiptop pots
- Recipes for hands and nails
- Male nails

No more chips

Reasons for nail varnish chipping or peeling are:

- the nails are not de-greased properly
- a base coat or top coat has not been used
- the nail varnish has been applied too thickly
- not bevelling to seal the edges of the nail – when the nail splits back, the varnish goes with it.

Tiptop pots
Storage and care of varnishes

What we expect from a nail varnish is that it:

- goes on smoothly, without streaking or separating
- covers the nail well without needing more than two coats
- isn't too thick or too thin
- dries quickly
- is hard wearing, and doesn't chip or wear off the ends of the nails too soon.

To keep a varnish at its best you should:

- keep it away from heat or sun, as it will thicken
- replace the top immediately after use, as the air will cause the varnish to thicken
- clean around the bottle opening regularly with a piece of cotton wool soaked in either nail varnish remover or solvent
- add a few drops of solvent to thin it out when it has thickened.

Recipes for hands and nails
A treatment for dry skin

You will need:

- a small plastic bowl
- a spatula
- a small handful of salt
- cooking oil.

1. Mix the oil and salt in the bowl until it is just thick enough to scoop out without it running through your fingers.
2. Massage the oil and salt into the hands, paying more attention to the rough, dry parts of the hand. Do this for about two minutes on each hand.
3. Rinse the salt and oil off with warm water.

The hands should feel lovely and soft, and will tingle from the improved blood flow.

A treatment for stains

Stains can happen on the nails and fingers if a client peels and chops vegetables or does gardening without wearing gloves.

You will need:

- a small plastic bowl
- one lemon, cut in half
- a nail brush or toothbrush.

1. Clean and dry the hands.
2. Squeeze both halves of the lemon into the bowl.
3. Dip the brush into the lemon, then gently scrub in a circular action around the fingers and nails where the staining is. As lemon has a bleaching action, the staining will fade.

INFORMATION

Take care: salt and lemon will sting if there are cuts on the hands or the cuticles are sore.

Male nails

Salon treatments for men are becoming more popular. Manicures are especially popular as men like to look well groomed. The basic routine is the same – the only difference is that they tend to have their nails buffed instead of painted. Some men, however, do like a clear coat of varnish to give their nails a healthy shine.

Men who do manual jobs, such as car mechanics and builders, may have untidy and tough cuticles. They may also have a lot of staining to the nails, cuticles and under the free edge, so make sure that you have a very good cuticle remover.

INFORMATION

For men with tough and stained cuticles, apply the cuticle remover generously, then leave it on for a couple of minutes. This will give the active ingredient sufficient time to bleach out the stains and prepare the cuticles for further treatment.

 MEMORY JOGGER

Test yourself and see how much you can remember. You could include the answers in your portfolio.

1. List **five** contra-indications to manicure treatments.

2. Describe what is meant by:
   - free edge
   - matrix
   - nail groove. ▼

MEMORY JOGGER

3 List **four** things that must be included on a clients' record card.

4 How do you decide on the shape and length of a client's nails?

5 List **six** fingertip facts.

6 How do you safely cut a nail?

7 What is the purpose of carrying out a massage on the hands and fingers?

8 List the reasons for using a base coat and a top coat.

9 Describe **six** points of homecare advice for a client after a manicure.

10 Describe **six** hygiene points when carrying out a manicure.

11 Give **two** different ways that you can set up for a manicure.

12 What is the difference between a male and a female manicure?

13 Give **two** do's and don'ts for varnishing nails.

14 List **three** points to think about when choosing a nail varnish.

15 Draw diagrams to show the finger rotation method of painting.

Section 5
EVALUATION

Self-evaluation

During your learning, it is important that you think about your progress, performance and satisfaction. The easiest way to do this is:

- to ask your client to complete a short questionnaire after her treatment
- for you to complete a *self-evaluation*.

These would be useful to include in your portfolio to show:

- that you are thinking about your work and maintaining good standards
- that you care about your client and are interested in her feelings.

When you go over and assess your performance.

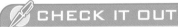
CHECK IT OUT

Before you begin, it is helpful if you and your tutor complete the following form, which details your first thoughts and feelings, and how you manage your time.

FIRST THOUGHTS

Name ....

1 How did you feel on your first day of the course?

....
....
....

2 Write four sentences about yourself and why you want to work in beauty therapy.

....
....
....
....
....
....

3 What do you think you will enjoy most? (It will be interesting to look back and see if you changed your mind by the end of the course.)

....
....
....
....

4 Do you always hand in work on time, or do you hand it in late?

....

5 Can you think of any ways that would help you to manage your time better?

....
....
....

Evaluating your treatment

CHECK IT OUT

Design a questionnaire about yourself and your treatment, to complete after every treatment. Think about what questions you need to ask and what information you need to include.

Here is a quick checklist to help you.

- Did you feel nervous?
- Did you feel that you carried out a good treatment?
- Did you talk about acceptable topics?
- Did you keep to your commercial timing?
- How much help did you need from your senior therapist?
- Were you well set up and organised?
- Were you and your client comfortable during the whole treatment?
- What did you find difficult?
- How good was the finished result?
- What could you have done better?
- Any other comments?

Client feedback form

The last questionnaire (on page 167) deals with how happy the client is with her treatment. Although we usually avoid asking a client closed questions with 'yes/no' answers, it is better to ask these questions at the end of a treatment. This is because it does not take the client too much time and effort to answer them.

TREATMENT EVALUATION

NAME .... DATE .... TUTOR ....

CLIENT NAME .... UNIT ....

Did your therapist introduce herself well and make you feel at ease?	Yes / No
Was your therapist's attitude towards you and your treatment good?	Yes / No
Did she carry out your consultation politely and confidentially?	Yes / No
Did she ask what your aims were for today's treatment?	Yes / No
Did your therapist explain your treatment to you before starting?	Yes / No
Did your therapist keep you informed of what she was doing at regular stages throughout the treatment?	Yes / No
Were you satisfied with the standard of your treatment and did it meet your aims?	Yes / No
Where you given useful homecare advice?	Yes / No
Did your therapist ask if you would like to book again?	Yes / No

What is your opinion on the products used?

....

....

Would you like advice on other treatments and products? If so, which ones?

....

....

Did you think that any part of your treatment could be improved? If so, how? (Suggested comments: preparation, organisation, surroundings, lighting, noise and the skill of the therapist.)

....

....

I would like to thank you for completing this questionnaire because it is an important part of my portfolio evidence.

CLIENT SIGNATURE ....

STUDENT COMMENTS

....

....

STUDENT SIGNATURE ....

TUTOR SIGNATURE ....

Index

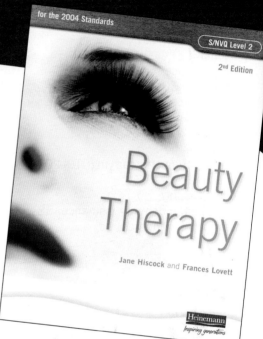
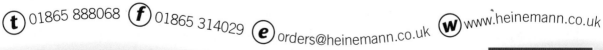
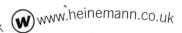
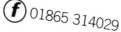
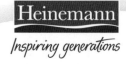